THE NO ONE GIRL

Rebecka Eden-Bond

First published in 2025 by Notebook Publishing, an imprint of Notebook Group Limited, Arden House, Deepdale Business Park, Bakewell, Derbyshire, DE45 1GT.

ISBN: 9781913206208

A CIP catalogue record for this book is available from the British Library.

Typeset by Onyx Publishing of Notebook Group Limited.
Front cover photography by LeSauvage.
Back cover photography by Rebecka Eden-Bond.

NOTEBOOK
PUBLISHING

This is a true story.

Some names of those described in the events included, or the names of places, have been changed or omitted for security purposes in order to protect the identity of the characters.

1
Out of Place

D O YOU EVER THINK ABOUT how you came to be where you currently are in life?

Well, this life—one that the luck of the draw had chosen for me (but that is okay, you know; we all have to deal with the hand that we are dealt)—begins partially in the early years of my life— which, if I'm being honest, I would rather not tell you about, as who wants to know about a perfect stranger's childhood, unless it's incredibly fascinating (which—spoiler—mine was not)? We've all had one, after all, and I never, on any occasion, feel the need to mention mine.

However, a little of it must be told here, you see, since some of the helpful traits that helped me to survive the traumatic experiences of my adulthood were partially formed during my developmental years, and my early years became part of the reason behind why I came to endure such experiences in the first place. With this in mind, I must allow you into this, my early life.

Although that part of my life might seem shocking, be assured that anything unpleasant that I experienced then paled into insignificance in the wake of that which lay ahead in my adulthood.

My early life is not something I have ever dwelled on and rarely think about; its inherent gloominess is contrary to my sunny nature! It was grim, yes, but I have never let it define me in any way.

Growing up in the middle of England on the outskirts of something of a forgotten-about city —albeit a most historical one— which has some very quaint looking parts to it, sharply contrasted with the depressing and run-down parts of the area—my early years but, in particular, adolescence, were spent almost entirely in poverty, around some deeply unpleasant people.

I recall this as a constant 'greyness', as feelings of gnawing hunger and cold, and generally depressing circumstances.

Though I came from poverty, moderate affluence was all around me in the immediate area in which I lived and there were many very comfortable large attractive houses there, with sprawling lush gardens and they seemed to have a peaceful atmosphere to them.

The house that I grew up in with immediate family, where I was the only girl, was very different to those nice homes. Dreary and with a very chaotic, most often aggressive, environment, it was nearly always full of men who possessed certain personality traits that were far from pleasant. Nobody was particularly abusive in their behaviour towards me when I was a small child, and that part of my life wasn't so bad.

Later, when I entered into adolescence, however, many of those around me began to treat me with utter contempt for growing into a young lady, as my appearance began to change and look very different, and I found myself to be the daily target of unprompted and disturbing outbursts from others.

The many male friends of the family, aged around nineteen to the early forties, often openly mocked my developing self and being that they would do so always in front of others, and as the shy teenager that I was at the time, I would feel my face become flushed with embarrassment at their comments.

They believed their behaviour towards me to be funny and clever, and, with no one wishing to defend the honour of a shy, slightly built, lone teenage girl, I had no choice but to stand and listen to their depraved insults, as I was constantly ordered to do as I was told. I was often made to act as a sort of servant for everybody and was expected to jump to attention and carry out any orders that I was given, while never answering back. On one occasion, while as usual having to fetch and carry for them, one of the men threw a one-pence coin at me and, in front of his audience in the room full of others like him, told me, 'There. Go and buy yourself something nice. That's all you're worth.'

Some of their behaviours were repulsive. Often, if the toilet was occupied, the men would stand over the bath, occasionally two at a time, and urinate into it. This left a stain, which I was forced to clean up, doing so while retching with revulsion.

It may surprise you to learn, however, that the degraded teenage girl of then did not grow up to possess skewed views of men; to the absolute contrary, I was never going to allow the behaviour of those who treated me badly to cloud my affectionate views or warmth towards others. I knew later in my teens, that such behaviour is not representative of the many good, lovely men. Thus, I have always believed in a balanced view of the sexes in that both matter to me just as much and I adore them equally.

During my adolescent years, the more I grew into a young woman, the more the hatred towards me from many of those around me also grew, not just from many of my peers but also, from some men and women. Their degrading comments were often accompanied by a slap in the face or grabbing and crushing my wrists and hands in an attempt to break them for being 'weak'(the perceived 'weakness' being based on having a soft voice and gentle nature), these being some of the sadistically controlling and degrading tools of choice of the adults.

Speaking in any capacity was received with anger, let alone daring to have an opinion. I was, therefore, a very withdrawn, and terribly nervous teenager who harboured a feeling of being most insignificant indeed.

Nothing in my adolescence felt as unbearable as my school life: abject humiliation was used as a tool to unnecessarily keep me in my place, both where I lived and at school. My schooldays during secondary school were ones that I would rather not dwell on, having been mercilessly and violently abused throughout their entirety for possessing the vulnerable combination of being very poor, very gentle in nature, and, apparently, so I would be told later, sort of ethereal looking, and completely alone. Being kicked, punched, and grabbed by the hair were daily occurrences, and were alternated with being pushed down the stairs, seemingly prompted simply for existing. 'Why don't you just die?' said the very angry leader of one of the main gaggles of loud-mouthed girls.

Though a few of the same boys constantly treated me violently, some other boys were kind and a few of my peers were, at times, sweet to me. The main instigators of my abuse at school were girls in groups. They rarely said or did anything to me when alone (a pattern that I would come to observe later in life: such people are usually cowardly without support).

My back was a favourite spot on my body for those wishing to beat me, whether from people my own age or adults, as they would approach me from behind and strike me until I hit the floor before then continuing with their beating. A kick was rare, but it happened on occasion, including a couple of separate incidents where I was kicked in the head by my peers, leaving a painful, large, reddened swelling on my forehead that everyone noticed but chose to ignore and not investigate. This was as painful as being subjected to what was termed as a headbutt, of which I excruciatingly was given a few times and threatened with often.

Once, during a lesson at school, two very extroverted girls were chatting with a group of boys about sex, when the girls began to speculate over what my body might look like naked, with them then encouraging the boys to grab me when I walked home from school and strip me of all my clothes, which the boys excitedly concluded to do later that day, pertaining to carrying out something of a sexual assault. In terror, while the others were occupied, I asked the teacher to be excused to use the loo, saw my exit to safety, and ran for my life, sneaking out of school and cutting my knees and hands as I scrambled through brambles and hedgerows, off the main school route in order to get away unnoticed and protect myself.

I had to learn to try and outwit those who chased and threatened me, by developing mental agility, quick thinking, and perhaps in my being hardier to the natural landscape than they were. This wasn't at all about toughness, but rather that I so often had to try and find safety. I was sometimes left with no choice but to flee school, as the only means of protecting myself from the, often violent, abuse that I was subjected to.

The place in which I grew up was surrounded by rolling countryside that looked quite stunning in the summertime, though could be terribly harsh in winter. Here, I sought solace in nature, walking through the fields and being amongst the trees and flowers, which became a therapeutic escape. I was fortunate in that respect, living among all of the nice landscape that provided a sanctuary for me from my depressing situation.

In some parts of psychology, it is suggested that we form some coping mechanisms in early life that stay with us. Well, I guess this was a major one of mine. I would always seek out natural environments and would continue to do so for the rest of my life, as a means of managing highly stressful situations, particularly when they involved being around people who treated me in a similar manner to that in my formative years. The calming effect of doing so always feels therapeutic.

But for almost the entirety of my adolescence, I felt frightened and nervous, perhaps because of knowing that another episode of physical or verbal abuse would not be far away and that anything I said, or even my very presence, could prompt it. Most of the time, I was silent and withdrawn. However, there were occasions when I would pluck up the courage to try and let out some of the bursting creativity within me. I tried to use my natural sense of humour as a way of getting my abusive peers to see me in a more humane light— after all, people usually are not angry when they find something funny, or so we might expect. But this failed in this instance, as my wit just seemed to anger them more. In fact, the noticing by others of any good quality in me just seemed to make some of those around me angrier.

Despite what I was subjected to at school, I received an exceptionally good standard of education (for a state education that is). The high quality of such, particularly with English and literacy, encouraged my natural way with words and written expression. This was noticed by a teacher who felt that I had, what they deemed to be an 'exemplary' talent for writing. Some teachers encouraged me to enter whatever writing competitions I could, believing this could help me get on in life, but there was neither money nor resources for me to enter the major talent searches, so instead I was placed in those that were free and consequently very minor and not leading to anything except winning books as prizes.

But in any case, it is difficult to concentrate on one's studies when distracted by beatings and with a tummy that is rumbling with hunger. Food was very scarce, as there was often no money to buy any with, but in any case, my basic needs, including being fed, were not thought to be important (though the vast majority of my young life was that way, on the rare occasions when I was allowed to visit my grandmother—a stoic and witty woman who was one of the most mentally strong of ladies that you could wish to meet—though she had little herself, I was properly fed and taken care of when with her). At school lunchtimes, I would see other pupils pile into the dining hall for a meal or packed lunch, and I would look on, alone and hungry. Occasionally, I was provided with or earned the ten pence required for a bread roll but sometimes I went without anything to eat at all.

Some of my contemporaries thought my desperately deprived circumstances to be hilarious, even finding it funny when at times, I became slightly too thin due to malnourishment, and I would stay outside at break times to try and escape them. One such time, it was pouring with rain, and, with nowhere to seek shelter for myself and my rumbling tummy, I tapped on the school's entrance door, manned by a Prefect—usually a spoiled and loud girl (I would go on to observe frequently in life that omnipotence is often awarded to those who crave it)—and asked to be let into the building to escape the bad weather but was simply laughed at in front of her audience of friends, 'we don't want poor people in here,' she said and slammed the door.

Outside I remained in life—and I would never know how to push my way in.

Money—or, rather, the incredible lack of it—in turn served to create a huge divide between myself and those who I attended school with. Often, they could not comprehend how I could be so poor and shy and bestowed in shabby clothes, yet so nicely spoken. I was also almost always alone, meaning that I was a target for gangs of teenagers who thrived on causing me to suffer further. It was only much later in life that I would be told, through the wisdom of some in the field of psychology, that intense vulnerability, coupled with any kind of good qualities or attributes (whether aesthetically or from the soul), when presented together, can be, in the sense of being preyed on by some, a dangerous combination.

A lady involved in professional dance wanted to refer me to a prestigious leading ballet school as she had noticed that my physical form, physique and burgeoning skill as a dancer was suited for professional ballet (though I was told that I needed to build up my energy and physical strength, which they were unaware were actually lacking due to poor nutrition and sleep deprivation), commented that I possessed fine posture and natural grace of movement—attributes that those who abused me, both of my age and adults, had picked out as, what they perceived as faults, as part of a seeming list of them that was so comprehensive that I was perpetually wondering if there was anything at all that was likeable about me.

But it was of no consequence anyway that I was perhaps thought suitable to potentially one day train with a ballet company, for ballet school was the domain of those whose parents could subsidise the cost of the training and so despite how suitable a candidate I may have been as a prospective future professional ballerina, the funding for my training would simply never be present.

Where I lived, I was told on a daily basis how I did not fit in because of not only that very posture and form that had been so suitable for professional dance, but also because of my particular voice and shyness.

But for the most part, I had to learn to try and avoid all kinds of abuses from others—from both those around my age and adults alike. Thankfully though, despite being frequently sexually harassed, I was never molested.

In my adolescence, it seemed that not only was I showing signs of being promising as a student of the arts in literacy and dance, but also, surprisingly, perhaps in acting. On a couple of occasions, there was a sort of makeshift drama class, and I found this interesting; being given free rein to escape into a creative world was exciting to me. Then again, the performance side of things filled me with dread: not the actual delivery of lines or movement but rather, distinctly, I had a sense of terror surrounding receiving attention. Some of my peers loved being the centre of attention—even desperately needing to be—but, in contrast, I was so afraid of being noticed.

Some of the other pupils, a couple of whom were nice to me,

were stuck with the writing parts during such lessons, and although I did not dare to suggest my contribution (I rarely spoke unless spoken to), they took a peek at my writing and, deciding to use it, even asked for my input.

Then when it came to the acting parts, most surprisingly, the poor, shy girl's appearance as a performer prompted an unexpected reaction from at least one person.

'That was *really* good, Rebecka,' said the teacher.

The class was silent until one of the girls loudly stated, 'She's not the same as us. We are better than her.'

The teacher answered however, 'Have you ever thought that what makes her different is actually what makes her suitable for this kind of thing?

The teacher told me. 'You are *beautifully* spoken.'

'But she's poor!' cackled another of the loud, overconfident girls.

'That's got nothing to do with it!' retorted the teacher. She then turned to me and said, 'See me after class. I would like to talk to you.'

The other girls were both incensed and perplexed that I had been noticed for a talent, but what actually felt good was that some of the other pupils seemed to love my writing—and I had liked producing it.

'Have you thought about performing arts school?' the teacher pressed on. 'You're perfect for that, and it'd really help to build your confidence. You have talent, both with your writing and your voice; even the way you move. They would build on that to develop your skills. Is that something you'd be interested in?'

Trying to contain my excitement at such a prospect, I replied with a simple 'yes'. However, my enthusiasm immediately evaporated when she mentioned that performing arts schools are fee-paying.

'I don't know much about that side of it, but I understand it would be largely subsidised for you in your circumstances and that there wouldn't be much to pay. That type of schooling could give you a chance to shine,' she carried on cheerily.

But I knew that paying anything at all would be too much and that the mention of it would prompt shouting of, 'What makes you think that anyone would ever be interested in *you*? — a response delivered with rageful scorn at the mere hint of anyone noticing a quality in me or the possibility of helping me to progress in life. Hence, as soon as fees, classes, and support were mentioned, I knew that it would be a no-go: such things were viewed as luxuries that I certainly was not worthy of.

The fact was, I never stood a chance of achieving anything simply through a combination of whatever talents or qualities I was noted for or no matter how hard I worked; it would also take funding for my education and training, but I was always told that I didn't qualify for that. With no funding for ballet school or performing arts school—both of which being prospects I had been recommended for, and which would have transformed my quality of life and future—I was instead left to plough on alone through utterly miserable years of schooling, involving a daily struggle just to obtain enough to eat and stay alert enough to make it through the classes. This was coupled with my mostly not having appropriate clothing or footwear—particularly shoes without holes in them and warm clothes in winter, when my hands would sometimes turn red in colour from the cold—and not to mention the constant distraction of being punched and tormented all day long by other pupils.

Lack of sleep was a problem, too, and often resulted in my struggling to concentrate on lessons. Some of those around me tended to stay awake almost all night long, and would often explosively argue into the early hours, or, if I had managed to go to sleep, I would sometimes be woken and shouted at, so I was never able to sleep properly due to this. But I knew that this was not a normal way of life or behaviour, as I always had a good sense of what it was to live healthily and as a peaceful person, I craved to be around normality, civilized people, and some loveliness.

Some of those from where I came from held views that were depressing and insular. I loathed being around those who were obnoxiously overly opinionated and of closed mind; those who made life unbearable for anyone who did not agree with them and who enjoyed humiliating people for no reason. It was behaviour that I would, for the rest of my life, find extremely difficult to abide. Unfortunately, however, I was surrounded by such personalities, and I longed to free myself from their ever-present wrath. Those people ruled my life back then and I feared them almost every moment of every day, but I would much later come to realise exactly what they were, all with the same mindset and belittling rhetoric in their stunted world.

Not all of those where I lived were unpleasant though: there were some nice people too. A few were kind to me on occasion, welcoming me into their homes.

I found that when I had the rare chance to be around those who were balanced and kind, from all walks of life, I began to bloom, but I grew up around an unconventional mixture of the educated, civilised, and lovely of both little or well-off means and then those who lacked true intelligence (though they considered themselves to be most intelligent indeed) or decency and who had unbalanced personalities to say the least (at the time, I didn't know exactly what they were, but only that I was afraid of them); the latter category there being unfortunately overwhelmingly more of. They would start trouble just by walking past them, disagreeing with them or even, as was often the case with me, just by my sitting alone reading a book (to aggressively point out how weird they thought that to be). It would take me many years to realise that there can be some who create chaos around others in this respect with their behaviour because they are unable to sit quietly with themselves.

Being beaten into submission for the way that I looked, spoke and walked and for my shyness meant that I yearned to be able to express myself creatively and to not have to completely play down or hide my possible creative abilities.

But it had been instilled in me that any good qualities I might possess, no matter if in what aspect of myself, should be hidden or apologised for. To add to this, I was rigidly told to never listen to my instincts as they would always be wrong and the opinion of others would always be right, and that I should unquestioningly do as I was told by everyone irrespective of how badly they treated me, as well as it being my sole purpose in life to make everyone happy (warped views that I would later learn suited others' need for control).

Perhaps you might wonder, in all of this, why no-one intervened to protect me? Well, I do not have the answer to that. Quite often, for whatever reason, people 'turned a blind eye' to it all, though were sometimes sympathetic. But crucially, I do not feel blameful towards anyone whatsoever, so I have never felt a need to question the reasons why. Nor do I wish to villainize those who were responsible for me. Moving forward from it all and achieving something good with my life was always the way that I wanted to go, rather than dwelling on the misfortune of my beginnings or blaming others for them.

From my mid-teens and during my development into a young woman, I was rarely called by my actual name, whether at home, school, or the area in which I lived; rather, I was instead referred to by some degrading term or another, including most often variations of 'bitch', with 'stupid bitch' (a term that was used frequently where I grew up, by both men and women, to, bizarrely, describe, almost any female who might be perceived to have some kind of appealing quality about them) in reference completely to my insignificance, not my intellect, being the most commonly used one (along with the particular girls and women who called me 'ugly bitch'). As an intensely shy, well-mannered and respectful girl, this was a strange choice of moniker—but that certainly did not stop it always being spoken as hatefully as possible.

Of course, teachers never referred to me in this way, but for the most part, they were the only people I knew, apart from some relatives I saw every once in a while, as well as a few of my peers at school who were nice to me and a few lovely people in the area who I occasionally encountered, who did not call me by this term of belittlement. It is possible that knowing these amiable people and the normal, friendly way in which they treated me, helped to mitigate some of the effects of the abuse that I was subjected to.

On one occasion, upon my leaving secondary school, a couple of months after turning sixteen, and having had a very successful interview for a performing arts course at college that I had been recommended for (only to be told days later that I didn't meet the criteria for funding for the course, so I wouldn't be allowed to attend), where to my complete surprise, I had been told by some of the tutors that I had met there that they thought me to overall possess all the right qualities necessary for possible success in the arts, I suddenly felt a surge in confidence: highly skilled, intelligent, professional people believed in me and wanted to give me an opportunity! In that moment, I experienced a strange feeling of excitement at the thought of my perhaps being about to earn myself a bright future.

Well, buoyed with this news and an unfamiliar feeling of happiness, I walked back up the street to the house that I lived in, only to find a group of local men who frequented the house standing outside its gate, loudly chatting to each other. I felt, as usual, very nervous and intimidated at the sight of them. But on this occasion, I must have been somehow showing slightly more confidence and slight happiness than normal in the wake of the promising news that I had just received.

The men caught sight of me and became quieter as they stared at me walking by. As I walked past them, one grabbed me by the arm and yelled, in their particular manner of speaking, 'Don't go thinkin' yer' somethin', stupid bitch,' and delivered a sharp slap to the left side of my face.

My legs almost buckled with the shock of the humiliation as my moment of happiness instantly evaporated and I reverted to being a quivering wreck. Any shred of belief in myself that I might have obtained at any time during my adolescent years was always immediately destroyed by those around me.

Having been classed as a psychologically normally developed adolescent, albeit an intensely shy one, the only legacy of my early life and the abuse and neglect that I experienced in my adolescence would be that, although I had developed an acute awareness of others' boundaries and wellbeing and was very sensitive to their needs and feelings, I distinctly did not protect my own enough and would often try to make myself lesser-than, so as not to anger anyone, and, as I would much later come to appreciate, I had been conditioned to just put-up with being abused.

History has shown us that some people's earlier lives have been truly tragic and far worse than mine, and it is for that very reason that I wish you not to afford me sympathy for my early life; I was simply one of others who were left to fend for themselves in most bizarre, degrading, poverty-stricken, or abusive circumstances, suffering at the hands of cruel people who had control over them at that time. I consider myself fortunate never to have endured any specific and acutely disturbing events in my early life, especially of the kind that others would later confide in me had appallingly happened to them or that they had witnessed in their early years.

But in terms of the deprivation and abuse that blighted my adolescent years, I have always viewed my start in life as 'that's luck (such as it was), that's life' and knew that I just had to get on with things as best as I could.

Certainly, coming from a deprived background can impede progress in the practical side of trying to do something professionally with one's life —in a dreamworld, it would be lovely if all whom are seen as having an aptitude or talent for something professionally, are given the same opportunities—but background in itself, at either end of the scale, has little to do with talent and strength of character.

Throughout my life, I have known people whose backgrounds range from poor and deprived, to the most comfortable, affluent, and highly prestigious. Nobody should be made to feel apologetic about the immediate world that they were born into, whether that world be one of privilege or one of deprivation. It just doesn't make sense to think otherwise, seeing as none of us have any choice in the circumstances of our early lives.

Well, I would rather not have even mentioned my own formative and adolescent years at all, if it were not for the fact that I would later be so categorized (very wrongly as it would turn out) by my unfortunate start in life and which would ultimately prevent my life from taking the progressive course that it should have done.

In spite of my unfortunate beginnings, I found that I had a natural affinity with many others. I had a real passion for so many of the elements that make life interesting: nature; music; travel; dance; fashion; comedy; film, philosophy, among others—all of which I would never lose and would ultimately shape me in the best of ways. I also had a thirst for knowledge which would never wane, always feeling that there was so much more for me to learn. Crucially, I was also greatly self-disciplined, and I learned to deal with the unpleasantness that I faced by focusing on the future and the possibility of nicer things. However, nobody would ever have known this just by looking at me; my strength was very much so a quiet, inner one.

As I became a young woman, I unwittingly attracted attention that I did not know how to deal with. I had a toned, proportionate dancer body shape with a distinctive arch of the back, a flawless porcelain complexion, large almond-shaped vividly green eyes, a symmetrical, heart-shaped face, and long golden-blonde hair. While this may read like a beautiful combination, I assure you that the reality to me was very different indeed and I certainly never thought myself to be beautiful at all; those around me saw my appearance as completely unacceptable, as they reminded me on a daily basis and so I did not feel good at all about the way that I looked.

I tried to avoid being noticed almost everywhere that I went locally. Wearing my hair loose or in plaits and with my pretty fashion style (customised by myself from hand-me-downs from the comfortably-off) would anger some women, who ordered me to wear boyish or downtrodden clothes and hide my hair. Sometimes, when I began to speak, my particular style of voice would anger them as well, so I was often afraid to speak in front of them.

What I did not know then, of course, was that the very aspects of myself that I was scorned for would be of such help to me to enter the professional arenas that I later did.

I did everything that I could to try and help myself and put all my efforts into working myself out of my situation.

While I was denied access to the drama schools and training in the performing arts by way of such criteria as not living in the right postcode or lack of local council funding for the arts, I was ushered into studying and working in sports therapy, because it was one of the very few courses on offer to someone with my potential skills in the area in which I lived. This was not at all what I wanted to do professionally but having been told that this was what I had to go into and with no chance of studying what I had been recommended for and what I really wanted to do, I had little choice but to go along with this instead, though I was grateful to be given any opportunity to progress in life. But after a year of training in this, the fully funded training ceased at the age of eighteen and one was then either expected to fund their own education with the help of their family, or else go on to be educated at university, where tuition was heavily subsidised and help with the cost of living was available. I was not sad about this in regard to sports therapy specifically, as it was something that I would never have chosen. But I would have very much liked to have gone on to study the things that I was passionate about and was recommended for. My higher education and the knowledge that I gleaned from it, however, was not wasted: I put it to good use in some small ways throughout the rest of my life, as it contributed to having some educated understanding of the mind and body.

With absolutely no assistance or study grants available as I was not eligible for them according to the tick-the-box application forms, and national scholarships or youth training programmes within the arts were practically non-existent in the area in which I lived, further professional studies would not be sustainable.

My writing was noticed by a lecturer of drama who I had an interview with and who allowed me to be granted access to a short English Literature course, having been advised that it might help me become a professional in the arts, as, he told me, 'Your talent will never be enough to be accepted to do that professionally without a relevant qualification'. But then I was told that the English Literature course would not be anywhere near enough and that I would need a degree in the performing arts to be allowed to work within them as a talent or performer, or, as a writer, to have my written works published for tv or film. So that was that.

I was ultimately informed that, though I had the necessary ability and, along with what was deemed to be a very good attitude to life, I did not fit any of the criteria for the funding required for any of the courses within the arts, partly due to the fact that where I lived I did not fall into any catchment area that was allocated for funded training or for any of the performing arts schools that accepted me. Neither was I eligible for sponsorship or a study grant as, besides the catchment area issue, there were seemingly only two other categories: you were from enough privilege to have help to self-fund your studies or otherwise it was always taken as a given, for some reason, that someone from my background of being very poor and neglected would surely be a delinquent who had misbehaved and broken the law and so, because of that, would be seen as deserving of a second chance, leading to those who fitted that description being given scholarships and study grants. So, being well-behaved (I would never have dared to step out of line in any way but, in any case, I wanted to live my life peacefully and without causing bother to anyone), I was never given my first. Not having the same opportunities meant that this was something that would continue for the rest of my life.

Therefore, in my desolate, solitary, circumstances as a teenager, it was impossible to fund the cost of studies myself, even while trying to earn as much money as I could in my situation.

One genial and helpful lady who worked in assisting the students at a college who had enthusiastically accepted me on a drama and performing arts course, seemed very frustrated that I was not eligible for any funding for my studies. She passionately tried to argue my case with the relevant local government departments, as she called around on the phone to anyone in a position to help allocate the funding for my studies that was automatically provided to almost everyone else my age, to allow me to become a professional within the arts and entertainment industry. But she was told that nothing could be done. 'I feel like I've failed you', she told me, 'I can see *so much* potential in you. You are a wonderful young woman, and I can see you *really* being able to achieve something as a creative person. You're perfect for the course and have the recommendations but I just cannot get around the funding criteria. Most young people are allocated grants or have help from their families to meet the costs of their studies – you are one of the most in need and deserving of help to get you on your way to doing something great, but I'm prevented from helping you'.

I thanked her for her efforts and reassured her that it was not her fault.

'Couldn't you move to somewhere that you might fall into the catchment area for funding?', she asked.

'I would love to do that and if the offer was there I would be so grateful', I answered', 'but that would take quite a bit of money initially and I don't have it. Anything I can earn right now would not be anywhere near enough to fund the initial cost'.

She looked very concerned; 'what will you do Rebecka?', she asked.

'I really don't know', I quietly answered, feeling completely downhearted, 'I am trying as much as I can to help myself progress. I will just have to continue to do so'.

My place in the world, as had been noted and encouraged by those professionals within it, seemed to be in the arena of performing with dance and my voice, perhaps a little in front of the camera and also publishing writing, but there was simply no funding for me to access any of these aspects of the arts professionally. I never qualified for financial study assistance, no matter how many funding or scholarship programs I applied to or how many professionals wrote letters of recommendation based on what they saw as my suitability. Funding for training in the arts was designated somewhat differently back then, especially in the area where I lived. As I did not fall into the categories on any application form by way of either my postcode or my circumstances, I was completely stuck in a situation where I was being urged to use the abilities that were kindly apparently seen in me in the interviews and auditions for drama school or a performing arts course that I had been recommended for, but ultimately being told, each and every time, 'Sorry, you don't qualify for funding for your professional training'. Ironically I was told that I had what was deemed to be raw talent (as others, of course, have also), but that I would not be allowed the training that would enable me to do something professionally with that.

Frequently walking for many miles to attend interviews and work, with a lack of good footwear, would sometimes cause my feet to bruise and bleed. There were no charities or organisations to help a girl like me: I did not fit into any category that qualified for that. Help simply was not available for me and so I resolved that I must therefore learn to live without it. Though I was often noticed in a very complimentary manner, I was never offered the help that nearly all of my peers seemed to be readily provided with. So, I tried to continue to make my own way in life and do as much as I could to help myself.

With no support of any kind and no way of funding further

studies, I had to accept that what I was apparently meant to do in the arts, in the professional opinion of those who saw some kind of suitability for that in me, was not going to happen.

Sadly, occasionally, young people can have what the experts see as much potential with a talent, skill or quality, and yet they will remain unseen simply due to circumstance—whether that be geographical location of where one lives, lack of funds, or no support from others. I was one of those such potentially accomplished young people who 'slipped through the net' for all of these very reasons.

Practical issues were holding me back terribly. With no funded scholarships in the arts available to me and in such deprived circumstances, I was utterly stuck. My career and training options were also limited to the area where I lived, which I longed to get out of so that I could broaden my horizons, but I had no money with which to leave.

On a couple of separate occasions, I was approached by a model scout while walking through a city centre. I had never thought of myself in that way but agreed to have a chat with them at the agencies to see if it could lead to my earning more income. However, whilst the women at the agencies telling me to 'invest in' lots of shoes and accessories for shoots, should any particular items not be provided on them (all standard back then when beginning modelling), along with expecting me to fund travel expenses to get to castings all across England several times a week until I was paid many months later for my first booking, may not have been a big deal to them, it very much so was for me; I never had enough money even for the bare essentials, no matter how hard I worked, because I had none of the support that most other young people receive, usually from multiple sources.

I worried terribly about how I was ever going to get out of this situation.

'It's alright for you,' I was told by an acquaintance one day, when we were discussing our struggles to get out of where we had come from. 'You're well-spoken, and people notice you. You'll have no problem getting yourself a good life.'

But it would prove to be far from as simple as that: though I was always acutely aware that I was not owed a nice life, sheer misfortune would come into play on a scale that I could not have imagined.

I did not know back then, just how horridly, bizarrely difficult my life was going to become in adulthood.

2

The New World

WHAT WAS THIS AWESOME NEW world that I had fallen into? As a sixteen-year-old, I had discovered the fashion, music, and nightclub scene, and now, three years later, I was immersed in it. It was the late nineties, and some cities in England were buzzing with a feel-good, happy-love vibe.

As both a dancer and a musical person, dancing and music were essential parts of my life. I had heard some of the DJs of the moment on the radio a few years earlier and been rather transfixed by their work: there is an understated artistry to it when done in a way that connects profoundly with the audience. Because of this, though I am not sure if they know it or not, many of the DJs at the time, with the vibe that they created, provided a temporary escape from the difficulties in our lives for those of us in awful circumstances. The pure house music at the time was uplifting, but there was also a blend of musical genres, such as funk, soul, and disco.

My musical tastes have always been eclectic: I adore orchestral arrangements just as much as a great house track, and, in fact, I had always felt that the two often marry together beautifully. I fell in love with the sound of an orchestra, including watching them perform and feeling the sound in person. I played piano a little and began to learn how to mix music. However, my circumstances meant that I never had the resources required to commit to learning the art of music as a professional or to sustain getting to know anyone in the music business properly. Sometimes I would watch the musicians and DJ's using the audio equipment and musical instruments, observing the ways in which they connected with their sound. Although I never managed to do anything musically due to lack of resources, my passion for music and its powerful ability to unite, move, and lift people's moods never faltered, and would forever stay with me.

From a young age, I was aware of the rhythm and timing of music, but also the power and style of vocals, even when spoken.

'You have a great speaking voice. Maybe we could get it sampled onto a track sometime,' I was told on a night out by a friend of an acquaintance, who worked in the music industry.

Recording semi-spoken vocals for a track would have been great, though this never actually got around to happening as I had no idea how to market myself in that respect. Rather, I would always wait to actually be invited because I thought that was the polite thing to do. But the mention of my speaking voice being good enough for professional recording from someone of the music industry did at least give me some inspiration for perhaps using my voice professionally.

Although it was not a popular view at the time—especially amongst those who regularly enjoyed nights out on the club scene— I did not like to drink much alcohol, and I was *completely* averse to the drug-taking that was so prevalent. If others took part in that, it was their choice and I would never lecture anybody—but I refused to get involved with what they were doing, even when I was mocked for this. I always wished to protect my health, both in the physical and mental sense, and live a healthy lifestyle.

I never interfered with anyone else's choices. They could do whatever they liked; it was just that it was not what I wanted to do. Not everybody wanted or needed to get high or completely drunk, or to be the loudest person in the room. For those like me, people could adore being in one another's company and want to hang out with an individual while still simply being themselves because they were vibrant or chilled out.

The venues that attracted amiable people who just wanted to have a good time by sharing a brilliant atmosphere and great music, were where I wanted to be. Those managing such places often wanted models and dancers with a stylish look in their establishment to add to its vibe, and, despite being very poor and shy and of no significance whatsoever, I was stunned to be welcomed into this category—which was fortunate, or I otherwise would have hardly ever been able to afford to get in.

My creativity became my form of expression. And right then, at that time of the 90's, expression in style was the thing—and I loved it. A fashionable older acquaintance in her twenties who had come from a comfortable background, had the good heart to notice how deprived I was, and I virtually nearly fainted with delight when out of the blue she gave me a few pieces of her no-longer-used stylish wardrobe, accompanied by a copy of a *Vogue* magazine. It was an act of kindness that meant so much to me. Perpetually, I dreamed of owning more clothes, but I could never afford to have more than a few items of clothing and just the one pair of shoes.

The fashion of the moment was exciting for both girls and guys. For me, my desire to dress nicely would never be about labels or showing off (I have always found that to be in bad taste), it was simply that having been prevented from owning many clothes at all or dressing in a nice way and also being a creative, I just enjoyed self-expression through dressing. The styles at the time did not necessarily have to be dressed up, either: they could be laid-back, almost effortless and lots of people made them their own.

There was something of a desire among many too, to strive to do something interesting with one's life, regardless of background.

It is odd to think how the nightclub and music scene could be related to all of this, but at the time, it was: it was more like a movement; a revival; like in some other eras, a significant time for fashion, music, and culture—and many of us eagerly embraced it.

Sometimes people who got to know me a little—both girls and guys—would suddenly give me a hug when talking to me and on a couple of occasions declared, 'aww Beck, you're so cute!', and 'I don't know why you feel so bad about yourself. You're cool'.

My confidence grew in this world where I could express my creativity a little. The previous crushing shyness that I grew up with began to transform; I could never show off and some shyness would remain, but in the sense of being able to socialise and converse with others, I found that I was absolutely fine. I was uplifting in personality and had a very keen sense of humour and always had ease in listening to others about their passions, endeavours, happiness, or sadness.

But finally having some small outlet for my creativity could not change the practicalities of the situation that I lived in. As a quiet and unassuming girl who completely avoided any type of trouble, I just wanted to go about my life normally. But I was constantly under threat of being beaten and publicly shown up by the people who saw me as too different where I lived. I learned that entirely playing myself down was not only expected but was the only way to try and avoid a beating. If I walked past some of the women or girls in the streets and there was more than one of them, they would usually punch me in the back or grab my hair, while shouting abuse about my appearance, cackling, and clapping and cheering each other on in their abusive behaviour. I was once beaten so badly that, after being repeatedly struck on the back, I struggled terribly to breathe. I lay gasping in a heap on the floor as the young woman, who had been angrily shouting insults about my appearance as a seeming form of entertainment in front of her friends as I walked past, stood screaming over me.

They never missed an opportunity to loudly tell me—and anyone else present—how ugly they thought me to be and indeed, having to listen to that on a daily basis certainly made me feel dreadful about the way that I looked.

On one occasion, a psychologist who was visiting someone in the area, stared almost open-mouthed when by chance, he met me, and I was being aggressively verbally abused and ordered around as usual, with some people delightedly telling him how I was 'nothing', while I stood in obedient silence. He seized a moment when he could talk to me out of earshot of others, had very nice things to say about how I looked and spoke, and, looking deeply concerned asked 'why does a girl like you put up with this kind of a life?'.

Stunned at his concern and interest, he told me that it was okay to speak, so I simply gently answered, 'well, I don't think I am anything special. I do try to get out of here and to change my life but no matter how hard I work; I can't seem to get anywhere'.

He looked at me earnestly and responded, 'don't listen to what they tell you. Get away from these types of people and get yourself a better life'.

Occasionally, a couple of good people in the area also tried to give me advice, telling me to take no notice of how some others treated me, explaining that the aspects that I was singled-out for were very good attributes to have and could consequently actually lead to becoming, as they saw it, successful in life, 'and if you ever do, I will be really pleased for you. You've got to believe in yourself', one sensible and intelligent man said.

But such kind advice was not enough to get me out of my situation; I was badly in need of practical help in order to achieve that. Perhaps at that time I should have run away, as I so often contemplated doing, but I had nowhere and nobody to run to and absolutely no money with which to do so and I knew that would mean placing myself in even greater danger. But escaping from there was exactly what I constantly dreamed of.

The practicalities of my situation and being completely alone meant that I could not get out of the city where I lived—but eventually, leaving the immediate area where I had grown up was at least a step in the right direction. Emotionally, I left that harsh early world behind as part of my maturing into an adult and tried to forget all about those abusive people who had blighted my early life: I had far more interesting things to concentrate on, after all! There was a whole world of creativity, life, and culture out there for me to be a part of, and I was more than ready to welcome it.

However, at the time, I had no realisation of my own self-worth and so sometimes reluctantly socialised alongside people who were very unhealthy for me to be around; you know, the kind of people who enjoy putting you down for no particular reason. With no means of being around the emotionally mature and interesting people who might have taken me under their wing, I felt I had no choice but to put up with the behaviour of those who enjoyed humiliating me by pointing out all the ways that I did not fit in with their ideal of what was acceptable (and you wouldn't believe how boring and dull that ideal was!). Anyone creative or embodying any kind of a beauty, whether male or female, would instantly be intimidated and 'put in their place', by them.

Though I was a lost young person, I did, however, know what I wanted to do with my life. But I simply never had the means or support to improve it, no matter how hard I tried.

For a while, I had no proper place to stay, and though I was never homeless in the literal sense, this was a scary prospect for a shy girl who drew a lot of unwanted attention and had no one in her life to turn to for help. However, though I felt frightened at my displacement, I was determined to get myself out of this situation and I was self-sufficient in many ways, because I had to be.

From a young age, I developed life skills, such as being able to cook well, on the occasions where there was enough food to do so and having to be very resourceful with ingredients. I could also sew and customise clothing to a certain extent and could manage all household chores. So, I knew that I was capable of looking after myself practically and emotionally and could manage alone if necessary, if I could get the opportunity to earn more money, and could therefore afford to find a place to live and begin to establish a stable life for myself.

After meeting with those at the couple of modelling agencies that had taken an interest in me, I very briefly found myself in London to look into taking this further, intending that a bit of modelling would help to subsidise developing myself as a creative while there. After gathering together some of what very little money I had earned through the work I could get, including teaching aerobics and very low-paid modelling or dance jobs, I bought the train ticket required for the journey to the capital. I truly believed that I had bought the golden ticket; the access to my route out of the depressing, abusive place that I came from; the route that would take me to the better, more peaceful, interesting, accomplished life that I dreamed of.

Entranced by some of its glorious historical architecture, entertainment within the arts, fun nightlife and creative possibilities, I hoped to stay in London for the next few years. But then I discovered that no matter how hard I worked, I simply could not afford the cost of living there on my own. Many young people making their way into the arts or modelling shared apartments to manage the costs, which at the time would have been great for me, but, as I did not properly know anybody there, this was never an option.

Despite my not wanting to be an actress, as I just did not feel I had the skill for that, I was advised to enquire into attending a performing arts or drama school while in London, as according to some of those in the industry, while they felt that I had something appealing for screen and should try acting, if I did not want to do it for a career, it would still be most beneficial for me to professionally train in this way because it would bring out the skills that they saw in me for different aspects of performance and creativity.

However, I found that I was once again not eligible financially for training in the performing arts and that no study grants would be available because I did not fit into any of the categories for eligibility. It would be impossible for me to financially sustain the cost of the studies alone, as what I could earn at the time would never be anywhere near enough. Hence, it would not be possible for me to train further as a professional in these fields.

Although I had no desire to be an actress, professionals within the arts tried to persuade me to try acting, so, although I did not think of myself in terms of talent, I realised that I perhaps was competent as something of a prospective performer. The few performing arts establishments I enquired at had welcomed me, but, as was always the case, they could not help me at all with pointing me in the right direction of the financial side of the studies that I had been so recommended to undertake, as I did not fit into any category to qualify for such help — the help that all young people making their way into any profession, including within the arts, initially need.

I was stunned that respected and talented people in the industry liked me and I could hardly believe that they had noticed me at all. However, though I worked hard, was always polite and punctual and did everything I could to help myself, I could never progress any further due to circumstance, and it might have been because of how well I spoke and presented myself, that those professionals did not realise the severity of the situation I was in.

That situation was one that I did not know how to get out of, no matter how hard I tried: as a very young person, starting out in life with none of the means available to them that others of my age were provided with, no matter how hard I worked, I could not cover accommodation and basic needs—and *especially* not in London, which was where I was told I needed to be if I was to progress in the professions that I was being accepted for. The chance for me to earn more money was there, in some modelling and by way of progressing in the arts, but I hardly ever had the money needed for travel and expenses in the first place with which to access the opportunity and the work. It was a vicious cycle that I constantly found myself in. Other girls who were not from well-off families would use their extroverted (or, dare I say it, in some cases, perhaps manipulative) personality to get others to help them, blagging favours from photographers and acquaintances, but it was never within my own personality to be that way. Neither would I ever even consider using people for my own advantages to get me to where I could be, as I had seen others do.

It became apparent that living in London on my own was not at all viable financially and that I had no choice but to return to where I came from in order to avoid imminent actual homelessness. With nowhere else to go, I was devastated to be forced by circumstance to return to that dark place that had previously held me back. That place where I could never be myself, where I did not belong; where I often faced abuse, sometimes violently so, in depressing circumstances.

So much for that golden ticket.

I hoped that this would be a temporary situation and continued trying to do the work that I could get to try and help myself to permanently escape this type of life of intense hardship. But any meagre earnings would never be enough to do so.

As much as I enjoyed the creative process of modelling, I couldn't rely on that for an income, as I found myself often being messed around by the organisational and business aspects, particularly when it came to being paid and that was very little in any case.

Then there was the sometimes overly direct attitude of some of those within it, that I had to learn to navigate. One of my first conversations with someone in the modelling industry involved them wanting me to pose entirely topless, not even covering myself with my arms, but I would not agree to this. 'It's just photographs,' my teenage self was sternly told by a loud obnoxious man involved in the casting. 'Look, if you won't show your nipples, then *you* have got a *serious* problem.'

Like many other models just starting out in the business, I was also often ordered to rush to get to somewhere across England at a moment's notice and at my own expense for a casting.

Although these are obviously not at all serious problems compared to those of some other professions, the point is that sometimes, these expectations of young people with little to no means could be ridiculous. I was always well-prepared and ensured I made a booking or casting on time, but I found that some of those in charge of bookings—in both modelling and sometimes branches of the arts—would often only inform the model or artist the day before or just hours before the booking or casting (something that would never change), when it was often impossible to get there—so unless one could afford to live in London, it could be extremely difficult to progress as a model, actor, dancer, or voice artist, if one could not afford to live in London or commute there from some distance away. I remained polite about it all, but such unrealistic and impossible professional circumstances can create real difficulties for a struggling young girl, nonetheless.

Modelling is rarely a full-time job for anyone unless they are at the top of the industry tree, which I was absolutely not (only at its very roots, given my situation), and considering I did not have the finances or contacts to spend much time in the then-epicentre of modelling (London), I therefore did not get the chance to do much of it.

Having undergone whatever dance training I could manage to afford from the little money that I earned from working in fitness and as a model, after earlier being denied the funding for a prestigious ballet school), I was told that I was skilled enough to pursue the art professionally and I tried to get as many dance jobs as I could. The limited amount of ballet training that I had been able to access, all that I could afford, became an asset to me during these times, and I blended this with salsa and freestyle.

Although performing in front of a crowd might seem paradoxical to my shy nature, I always felt that the work is separate from me in that sense; as I would go on to see all aspects of this in the future, whether it be with my voice, written words, whatever, the spotlight is on the possible artistry that I create—and this way allowed me to be not so scared of the attention that I received for that possible bit of artistry. All that I knew was that when performing or producing something creative, I felt entirely connected with myself and with the audience; it felt like a certain and very profound sense of freedom. It was also the only outlet that I had to express the strong creative part of myself that I had nearly always been forbidden from showing.

But dancing was very poorly paid.

None of the different aspects of work paid much and I continued to struggle to earn enough for my basic needs.

My miserable circumstances, however, were not a reason for self-pity; I absolutely knew that I could entirely overcome them given half the chance.

However, despite the frequent compliments from industry professionals on—according to them—my abilities, pleasant attitude and look, and my hoping that the people saying these things to me would be about to put me on the right path to allowing whatever prospective talent that they so kindly saw in me to flourish, nothing would ever happen in terms of any opportunities. Perhaps they were simply unaware that I had never had neither the resources nor the backing others had to progress with whatever the potential was that they saw in me.

But as someone who had, despite being accepted and welcomed into this professional world, been repeatedly denied a place to train as a professional within the arts simply as a result of lack of funding, I unfortunately lacked all of the connections and credentials and help with guiding a career in the arts that a person usually acquires by attending a stage school or being well-connected, and, without the little pinch of help (that I certainly never expected from anyone but was in any case required) and tiny bit of good fortune needed, there was nothing at all that I could do to resolve this situation.

Of course, not exclusively everyone who establishes themselves within the arts has been to a stage school or has a degree in dramatic arts: some found their way as a performer by beginning in a local performing arts group for young people, a route which I looked into. But again, virtually all opportunities in this respect seemed to be focused on London, although if one lived in, say, Manchester, there were some youth training groups and sponsorship-style opportunities in the arts available there too, but where I lived, these were generally non-existent.

With the avenues into the performing arts, that I had been recommended for, now all exhausted through lack of funding, or simply not being in the right place at the right time, I realised that such training and opportunities in that which I had been selected for professionally were never going to happen.

One summer, I met a good looking, mysterious guy who also happened to be a great dancer. He barely spoke to me, although he stared at me a lot. He told me that he was on leave from his service in the military but was going away again soon on further active duty. To my surprise, he asked if I would write to him while he was away. Some months later we arranged to meet up. We went for drinks and chatted, and my being an enthusiastic listener, he seemed to find it great to get the opportunity to talk to an understanding female about himself. We discovered that we liked the same music and had very similar interests. Conversation between us flowed and I was delighted to hear about his travels.

It is not often that you meet someone with whom you share so many of the same interests. *How great is this to have found such a good friend with so much in common?!* I thought.

But soon he then tentatively told me of his strong romantic feelings for me, which took me by surprise. I soon fell for him too. He was knowledgeable and quick witted, and looked dashing with his shiny hair, good complexion, attractive eyes, and style of clothes (his smart way of dressing being, despite the poverty of his own early years and him not being of any wealth, simply due to his knack of knowing how to invest in clothes properly and how to style them well).

Ethan and I saw each other whenever he was home, and, when he was away, we would keep in touch.

He noticed straight away what happened to me when we would go out locally (this reaction was prolific where I came from but hardly ever happened to me in London, where people would kindly tell me that they loved my look); the aggressive questioning of the way I looked and walked by other young women, in groups, in the local nightlife venues.

Sometimes, when I returned from a modelling or dance casting, they would intensely kick it up a notch to let me know of my insignificance, as I would be confronted with their shouting and cackling. At such times, I would lower my head in embarrassment, while wishing that they would just leave me alone, as they loudly verbally attacked me with their spiteful-looking expressions, telling me in abusive terms how they found the way that I looked, dressed (an elegant dress, for example, could evoke fury in them for some reason) and walked (according to others, the ballet posture and perhaps slight runway-style gait, having been natural assets from a very young age and were probably, unknown to me, exaggerated by the professional training and bit of work that I did in this respect) to be completely unacceptable. They were no less scathing about the way that I spoke—my voice was naturally soft and feminine, and, through study of literature and the arts from a young age, my style of speech became gently moulded towards well-spoken neutral English. But many times, I was told that I didn't have the right to speak like that because of the city and poor background that I came from (by people who lived there). For my safety, I would often try to play down my appearance and the way that I spoke. Others would sometimes come to my rescue when it became obvious that I would be physically beaten but often I would simply leave a venue to get away from the hassle.

'You do realise that they actually know you look great. They just intimidate you because they resent you', said a guy, upon seeing me cower away from them, while another said, 'You're different and you stand out. That is what their problem is. Be proud of who you are'.

But I had never gone out of my way to be different and had always been self-conscious of standing-out. I also did not feel I had anything to be proud about. I had no idea how to cope with such reactions that made me worry over my behaviour and appearance, always thinking that it was me who was in the wrong and trying to correct whatever I guessed it might be that had caused the problem. I felt like an oddity where I came from as my appearance, demeanour, and the way that I spoke was near-constantly pointed out as being different to most others around me.

For the first eighteen months together, Ethan and I had no proper home and because he was working away most of the time, it was difficult to truly ground ourselves anywhere. For a while, due to circumstance, we had to live in a tiny room in a grim, house in a grim area, surrounded by narcotic drug use and all kinds of goings-on. It was very depressing indeed. My safety was constantly under threat and so I had to try and conceal my appearance as much as possible so as to be noticed less.

We saved to buy a home of our own as soon as we could, though could not yet afford to go further afield than the city that we lived in, but it would be an initial foot on the property ladder to eventually get us where we did want to go. We bought as best a property as we could afford, which was a small nineteenth century terraced cottage, as its diminutive size meant that the mortgage would also be small and therefore manageable. We had to have somewhere to live and mortgages for a house of that size cost the same as rent each month, minus the deposit. We knew that savvy investment at this stage, albeit by going without almost all material things as the only way that we could manage to achieve that, would set us up well for later on. We directed all the money that we had into buying the house, so much so that we were left with nothing to furnish it with. So, for the first couple of years, the house was without carpets, proper furniture or even a fridge and we didn't have access to a washing machine initially and so I washed all of the laundry, including some of Ethan's military uniform, by hand in the bath.

It was not the easy option by any means, and we only had each other to rely on, but our sacrifices meant that we were on the property ladder, in advance, despite both coming from highly disadvantaged backgrounds and with no help. We were willing to go without all comforts, a car, a social life, everything, in order to ensure that hopefully, we would never face the risk of being displaced again.

Meanwhile, for well over a year, I had been experiencing a

female health issue that I had never experienced before, in the form of symptoms of pelvic pain and bleeding (that was mortifying for me to say but there, I have said it).

I was advised to go to the hospital due to the symptoms of pain and bleeding where, in the absence of any obvious clinical findings, the doctor concluded that I must have some kind of chronic female-health specific issue, such as the onset of endometriosis, though there was no sign of this.

'You are far too young to have any serious female health problem,' the doctor told me, and I was thus discharged with no further follow-up.

I was now still suffering with pain and bleeding symptoms which had become fleetingly intense at times and on one of those occasions, Ethan insisted on taking me to the hospital again. In light of these symptoms, the emergency department doctor took some blood and seemed concerned as she told me, 'Your blood test results have come back showing that you have elevated white blood cells, which means your body's fighting something. I am going to admit you as an inpatient to see if we can get to the bottom of this.' (I would much later learn that the elevated white blood cells were possibly due to the irregular bleeding).

Whilst the doctor on the general medical female ward that I was sent to was kind, he concluded that there was no cause for concern, 'You're very young, so there's no need to worry about serious gynaecological disease. But I will advise your doctor to keep an eye on the symptoms.'

Sure enough, the symptoms did not go away, and so a few months later, I revisited my doctor, who found it to be highly unlikely that I had any serious or chronic condition. However, upon the advice of the hospital doctor, he referred me for my first Pap 'smear'—a cervical screening test. I thought little of it, and when my doctor told me that the smear test results were found to be normal, I was told to stop worrying, and, again, that no follow-up was necessary.

Over the following eighteen months, though I felt foolish in doing so, I returned to see the same doctor on a few occasions, as the symptoms were becoming very slowly, but progressively, more troublesome. However, the symptoms were not taken seriously, and this was not helped by my looking so young: at the time, it was generally thought to be impossible for very young women to develop anything as severe as gynaecological cancers.

By now, I was more frequently in pain in the pelvic area. During times of relief from the symptoms, I was able to function and get on with life. However, due to the painful symptoms, for the most part, I was beginning to find it difficult to manage consistently working and my dance training.

Around this time, I was recommended to a department that handled fashion and photographical features for a national Sunday newspaper: they were interested in shooting me for a feature and were hoping to launch a great model out of it. I was unsure about taking the newspaper people up on their offer, as the thought of being in a newspaper made me feel uncomfortable: my reservedness holding me back.

Ethan, on the other hand, was really encouraging. 'This could be a great opportunity for you.'

I explained to someone within modelling how the media was not my thing. The fashion and editorial magazines would be fine, I felt, but there was a different feel altogether to doing newspaper features. Referencing how a particular supermodel had started her career the same way, however, she then explained, 'Sometimes, it's simply the course of how a model's career takes-off. It's just a fashion shoot with a nice fun piece for the media group, not a trashy tabloid article. There's a difference.'

Well, I thought, *if it was good enough for a style icon and supermodel* (though of course I absolutely did not think I could be either of those), *then who am I to look down on such an invitation?* With this conclusion reached, I agreed to the shoot, and was sent a train ticket to travel to London to meet at the newspaper's headquarters.

I need not have worried about the shoot: the people I worked with that day were completely professional and lovely to me. The photographer came to meet me at the newspaper HQ and drove me to another building, where we were to do some of the shoot. There, I was introduced to the hairstylist and the fashion stylist I would be working with who were both also very friendly.

After changing into the dresses and bikinis that they had selected for me, I walked out into the studio. They all seemed pleased by my appearance.

'You really have star quality, definitely.' said the stylist, who often worked with celebrities. I blushed, finding such compliments incomprehensible; I felt most un-star like indeed. 'You have one of the best bodies in the business! All natural,' she continued in her kind enthusiasm, 'but it's just something about you. You just have that quality, and it shows when you walk into a room.'

I did not know how to respond; where I grew up as a teenager and then as a very young woman, I was always told, especially by other women, that I looked too different and did not fit in, and that this was completely unacceptable and was reminded often how completely insignificant I was thought to be. And now, professionals connected to the worlds of modelling and the arts and entertainment industry were telling me very much the opposite of things about myself!

'This will properly launch your career,' the photographer said. I was dubious about that as I did not believe that I could get far as a model, not least because there were of course some who were absolutely stunning and fabulous. Still, it was an opportunity that I had kindly been given to possibly go on to have a good chance of earning a decent living and I enjoyed the process of creating lovely images, so I was very grateful.

Out of the blue, the photographer said, 'Would you be a pin-up? You'd be a total sensation.'

The stylist exclaimed to the photographer, 'That would be such a waste of what she can be! She has an old-era Hollywood movie star look.'

'You might be right,' replied the photographer to the stylist. 'I was thinking of the male readers. They would love her.'

'I know I'm right,' replied the lovely stylist brightly as she arranged my clothes. 'We've got a totally natural, long-haired, long-legged beauty in front of us, *and* she's funny and likeable.' *Who was that?* I wondered as I looked around the room, thinking that someone else had walked in; *she couldn't possibly be talking about me.* The stylist continued, 'The men will love her anyway. And the *female* readers will love her, too.'

The talented photographer had a great sense of humour, and I felt comfortable and safe working with him. This newspaper photographical stuff was a less-than-ideal scenario for what I wanted to do with my life, but the photographer put me at ease, and it was only a fashion shoot and fun feature for a Sunday newspaper, so no big deal.

When we had finished the studio shoot, some location shots were required, and the photographer drove me and one of the other people working on the shoot, a funny and mild-mannered guy in his late twenties, to an apartment building in the London docklands to get some varied images. But after only a few more shots were taken, to my embarrassment, the pain symptoms started again. I excused myself for a moment, as feeling faint, I arched over, my arms wrapped around my lower abdomen, the sharp pain gripping me.

That was how the symptoms would often happen, at the most inconvenient and unsociable of times. I had felt a little of them coming on during the journey to London and had arrived at the publications' studios looking a bit pale and lethargic, but it had not seriously impacted my ability to be a consummate professional until this moment.

I had to confess to the shoot team that I did not feel well, though I did not tell them of the pelvic symptoms, and the photographer commented that I indeed looked 'peaky'. Thus, we decided to call it a day, having obtained enough shots for the features team to look over.

The photographer kindly offered to drive me to the train station. On the way, he had to stop at a shop for an errand and asked if I wanted anything from there to help me feel better. I responded that I was fine, thanks, but when he returned, he handed me a sweet drink.

'For some energy for the journey back,' he said.

When we arrived at the train station, I was still feeling faint and struggling with the pain. The photographer seemed concerned over whether I would be okay with getting home, but I said that I would be fine. I thanked them for being great to work with; the photographer had not had to go out of his way like that to look after me on the shoot, but he had, nevertheless and that was kind of him.

I thought no more about the shoot or feature but when a couple of months had gone by, and none of the shoot had appeared in print, I began to worry that I might not have been professional enough or had not produced good enough images, so I called the people who were handling the feature to politely check that I had properly done what they had asked of me.

'Your pictures were great; we loved them,' I was told. 'We were putting the feature together ready for print, but plans then changed: after your shoot, our new lady editor decided to take things in a new direction with the newspapers image, so we won't be featuring models and fashion shoots now.'

It was the editor's publication of course and she had the right to do whatever she felt was best with it, so she had done nothing wrong at all in making that decision. I just accepted it.

But although I was nervous about the publicity aspect of the shoot and feature, I had been buoyed by the prospect of all the work that I was told would come from it. 'Lots of great opportunities are going to open-up for you from this', I had been told. Such opportunities, that I had so far been denied because of my deprived start, would have improved my life dramatically and allowed me to go on to develop myself with my creative work.

As disappointing as this was, missing out on all of the potential work that could have come my way as a creative, I had to move on from it as I had more pressing concerns with the frequent increasing pelvic pain that I was experiencing.

3
Unheard

JUST AS IT IS OFTEN awkward for guys to talk about their male-specific health problems, it is frankly somewhat embarrassing to me to have to mention my experience of my gynaecological cancer. I believe that it is usually good to keep personal matters just as that: personal. Nevertheless, I have to make mention of it being that what I have survived in terms of my female specific-type cancer is the reason why I later came to have some disturbing experiences in society and miss out on doing anything good with the artistry that I was being told that I had and was urged to use.

The symptoms of pelvic pain and irregular bleeding were distinctly the only two symptoms that I would have and there were no others. Well, now, as these two symptoms—the pain being far the most severe of the two—became increasingly more persistent, I felt that something was not right.

These specific symptoms had begun very subtly, hardly noticeable at all at first, but were now increasing.

But although I was suffering in this way, I had no concern over having any kind of serious illness, as I had believed the doctors when they had assured me that everything had been ruled out in the previous tests. So, when my next cervical screening test (sometimes referred to as a pap test or smear) was due, I thought nothing of it and did not worry.

As before, the test results came back as entirely normal. 'You see? Normal!' my doctor said as he showed me the test result. 'You have no problems with gynaecological health.'

Tentatively, I tried to explain my confusion at this. 'But I have pain in my pelvic area, and irregular bleeding,' I replied politely.

'It's just a normal part of your cycle,' said the doctor. 'My dear, all that I can do is reassure you that you that this is not something to be concerned about.' He was nice and sincere, and so I accepted his words.

However, the symptoms continued, and some months later, after suffering a bout of severe pain, Ethan once again took me to the hospital at his insistence and there, I was admitted to a gynaecological ward.

The lead nurse refused to believe that a very fit, very young-looking girl could have any kind of a serious physical health problem. She scornfully demanded to see evidence of the bleeding. I showed her, but she simply snapped, 'it's just your normal female cycle. You are too young to understand it'.

She would not listen to my polite explanation of that, in fact, through my commitment to health, my academic education of physiology and being a dancer and athletic, I was completely in tune with my own body, and I was therefore very aware that this bleeding was not at all normal. Would she therefore please kindly reconsider investigating the symptoms? 'No, that's absolutely not necessary', she snapped before storming away, muttering about me being a 'silly young girl'.

Ultimately, given that the cervical screening results had been negative, it became very apparent that nobody was going to take my symptoms seriously at all, even on this gynaecology ward, and that they would not investigate the matter further.

For some strange reason, a psychiatrist then appeared at my bedside.

When he introduced himself, I assumed that there had been some mistake; that he had gone to the wrong patient or the wrong ward.

'I'm sorry; I think there's been a mistake,' I said. 'I'm here for gynaecological issues.'

'There's been no mistake,' he responded. 'I am here to see you, Rebecka. Will you come this way with me, please?'

I was puzzled; I had never had any psychological treatment or any issues of that nature, but because he was a doctor, I unquestioningly did as he asked, following him out of the ward and along the corridor to a side office where he closed the door and we sat down.

'Right,' he said with a grin, 'how are you feeling? How are your symptoms?'

'Well, I am not sure that I feel comfortable discussing them with you, as you are a psychiatrist, not a gynaecologist!' I answered humorously, trying to adopt a light-hearted tone. Pleasantly, I enquired, 'May I please ask what this is about? I don't understand why a psychiatrist wants to see me about my gynae problems.'

'I just want to ask you some questions,' he said, in a reassuring tone. He said this so benignly that although I found it odd that a psychiatrist wanted to assess me for anything at all, it did not feel like it was something to be hugely concerned about: I thought that maybe it was just routine to do this sometimes in hospital; part of a sort of wellbeing check. At least, that's how it seemed. So, when he said that he needed to find out a little of my background in order to help him, I allowed him to proceed with his questions. Number one: 'So, let's start at the beginning. Tell me about your childhood.'

I was bemused by this question; after all, it bore absolutely no relevance to the reason why I was in hospital. 'Why do you need to know about that?' I asked, politely.

He simply replied, 'It would be helpful if you just explain a little about your earlier life.'

I responded casually, 'I don't really see how. But, well, it was a bit grim, I guess, but I overcame it as an adult.'

Following his further probing, I answered his numerous questions about family, school life—everything, it seemed, that could possibly have featured in my upbringing, in the same nonchalant manner. He seemed to relish this questioning process and the answers that I provided, and, as a result, I began to get an uneasy feeling surrounding the situation.

'Can I please ask what relevance this has to anything?' I interrupted.

'It will be helpful just to answer the questions, Rebecka,' he said gently.

'When you feel that you are having the pain and bleeding, do you think of a specific event in your childhood or adolescence?'

Suddenly, the realisation set in that it was being inferred that actually, the gynaecological symptoms were psychological. I responded softly, 'No, I do not. I don't think about my early years. It is not imagined pain and bleeding. What have the pelvic symptoms got to do with my early life?'

'Well,' he continued, 'when people have trauma during childhood, it manifests itself during adulthood in other ways.'

I quietly and politely answered, ' my formative years have left me tending to be a bit shy but I do not feel traumatised. Are you suggesting that I am imagining my gynaecological symptoms because my early years were far from optimal?'.

He ignored my question while looking down at his notes. 'Now, you have been weighed in hospital and found to have a borderline-lower end of scale BMI. How is your relationship with food? Do you eat normally?', he asked.

Confused by what relevance that had to do with anything, I answered, 'I eat healthily'.

'So do you restrict foods? Do you diet?', he probed.

I simply answered, 'I keep to a healthy diet'.

His face seemed to light up at this answer. 'So you like to stay thin! Do you think that you are a big girl? Do you feel fat?'

This is bizarre, I thought to myself. *Why the interest in my size?* Though slender, I was now not skinny and had a curvaceous shape and excellent muscle tone. My body, with the complete exception of the pain and bleeding symptoms, was overall very healthy indeed. 'I like to keep myself in good shape. Of course, I have to keep to a certain body shape for modelling and dance,' I answered.

Again, he seemed to ignore this information as he continued to write his notes. 'So,' he continued, 'do you ever make yourself vomit?'

Though puzzled by the absurdity of this questioning, I answered, 'No. I would never do that. I really like to look after my teeth; I would never cause damage to myself.'

Though I stated that I found the questioning strange, the Psychiatrist retorted that he thought it to be completely acceptable.

'I do not believe that the gynaecology department is suitable for you,' he said simply. 'Your childhood experiences combined with the reporting of physical symptoms that are non-existent means that you may need to be referred to psychology.'

Confused at his words, I softly replied, 'but, I have never needed or had any involvement from psychology. Apart from my reserved nature, I don't have issues from my early life that trouble me; I don't even think about it. *You* asked *me* about it—I did not come to you. Why won't you believe that my gynae symptoms are real?'

'Because the tests state that they are not. I am making a recommendation: that you are referred to the psychology department, where you will be assessed.'

I felt a flash of fear run through me and quietly responded with, 'I respect you as a doctor, but this is unnecessary.'

The psychiatrist did not answer and instead just stared in silence at me.

'Is this over now? May I leave please?' I asked. He nodded to gesture that I could.

The psychiatrist followed me out of the door and called for a nurse as I walked down the corridor to the nurse's reception where I asked to use the phone.

As I was dialling home, the psychiatrist spoke to the lead nurse at the reception, to discuss his psychoanalysis of me. 'She wants to go home,' I heard the nurse—the same one who had demanded to see evidence of the bleeding symptoms, though still not believed me even when she saw this—say to him, referring to me contemptuously and only by my surname. However, he responded that I should not be allowed to leave without a referral being done for a psychological analysis because, as he explained to her, 'Yes, the pain and bleeding is psychosomatic. I have established that she was from a deprived and abusive background, and so with the test results all being normal, I conclude that she is interpreting earlier emotional trauma as physical pain. She looks slim, as well, so an eating disorder could be her way of controlling early trauma.'

The nurses did not question what the psychiatrist said and now viewed me as wasting their time.

I called Ethan and told him what had happened. He could not understand why a psychiatrist had become involved with my care and thought they might have made a simple mistake but said he would come to the hospital.

Quietly, I sat on the hospital bed in a state of fear and disbelief; my gynaecological symptoms had been classed as psychosomatic (which basically means imagined) and because of that I was now being referred to a psychology department, for which 'analyses and treatment' had been mentioned.

When Ethan arrived, I nervously asked him, 'Why won't anyone believe me that my symptoms are real?'

The nurse told Ethan that the psychiatrist believed my symptoms to be psychosomatic and had advised that I was to be discharged from the gynaecology department altogether and had instead referred me to the psychology department. Ethan, perplexed, politely asked to speak to him about this but he refused to see him.

'This is not right,' Ethan gently insisted. 'Her symptoms are real; I *know* they are. I live with her and see her suffering. She doesn't need a mental health referral at all', he told the nurse.

But she said that there was nothing that she could do and that we would have to take it up with our doctor.

We did so, but upon receiving the letter of referral from the psychiatrist and listening to me state how strange this was when I had only reported gynae symptoms, the doctor simply said 'There is nothing I can do. I have to assist in the referral'.

'But she doesn't *need* this referral; she needs treatment for the pain and bleeding,' Ethan politely said.

'The gynaecological symptoms that she has been reporting have been diagnosed as psychosomatic,' the doctor responded to him. 'I'll refer her to the psychology team, as requested by the psychiatrist.'

'This might seem strange, but if I were you, I would go through the motions of it,' Ethan advised me. 'I would go to the referral appointment and show them how wrong they've got you; that you don't have issues from your childhood that are causing you problems, that your physical symptoms are real. Then, they will realise that what they're doing isn't right and give you the treatment you need for the pain and bleeding. I think they need to meet you properly and see who you actually are, rather than looking at things on paper. I'll come with you if you want me to; I'd like to tell them myself how wrong what they're doing is.'

This made sense, in a strange sort of way, so I tearfully agreed.

Fearfully, I attended the scheduled psychological assessment, accompanied by Ethan, but felt perplexed by the whole thing. it was held in a place that was mainly staffed by those from the department of psychology but was supported by psychiatrists. It was such a degrading place to go to and some of the staff seemed mystified as to why I was there, as it was made clear that I was very out of place. *What on Earth was I doing here?*

'I just want to leave. Please, let's just go,' I quietly begged Ethan.

'It's wrong that you have to go through this, but you need to prove to them that you're not imagining the symptoms,' he said firmly. 'I've seen things like this happen before, where a psychiatrist insists that they're right about something when it turned out that actually they've got it wrong.'

So, I very reluctantly stayed and had the assessment with a young female junior psychiatrist, whose role, apparently, was to assess me and assign me to a psychologist or similar professional for some kind of therapy or treatment, though they never stated what this was or why I needed it, especially given that I had never had mental health problems.

'So, you have been referred to us because of problems stemming from your abused and neglected childhood and symptoms of an eating disorder which are prompting you to imagine that you have pain and bleeding,' she said.

I felt exasperated at the extent of this misinformation, but gently explained, 'I don't have problems from my childhood or an eating disorder. The psychiatrist who came to see me on the gynaecology ward—who I still cannot understand why had felt the need to see me in the first place—asked me what my early years were like, and so I answered him honestly about them, in a matter-of-fact manner. But I don't have problems from them that really trouble me, and I never said that I did. Nor do I have any problems at all with anything related to my diet or any eating disorder. I do have pelvic pain and irregular bleeding, however.'

'Denial is common in these situations,' she said.

'Please, I am not in denial about *anything*,' I softly pleaded, 'I know who I am, and I would never think or behave in that way.'

And yet she just continued to ask questions on my childhood and adolescence, which she seemed to be most interested in dissecting.

She explained that she was doing this because it states in some parts of psychiatry that people from my kind of early years become poorly functioning adults.

Bewildered, I responded politely and softly, 'Not all such circumstances are the same. If you don't mind me saying so, that is illogical thinking. I have always taken personal responsibility of my own life and behaviour, and I choose to do the very best I can, regardless of my earlier experiences. I have never made my early life an excuse for anything.'

My individuality was not considered at all with this broad generalisation. Sure, I was struggling to achieve what I wanted to, having been held back by the practical side of having a deprived start in life, but I was doing the best that I could to pull myself out of that, was (I hope) respectful to others, and there were many things in my life that suggested that I had overcome and adapted to what I had been subjected to as an adolescent. But I was now being told that it was all futile because I had the simple misfortune of a deprived start and living around abusive people. I began to worry about this and question myself as a person; *what am I doing wrong?*

The junior Psychiatrist continued with her analysis of my background which included her assuming that because I was from deprived circumstances, I must surely be from a one-parent family, the worst-case scenario of an area, and probably raised by alcoholics. When I informed her that none of those assumptions were true at all, she expressed surprise.

Just as it had been with the hospital psychiatrist, the junior psychiatrist had, upon through their questioning by way of trying to figure out why I felt I had the symptoms of pain and bleeding, and consequently learning of my abusive and deprived upbringing, despite no mention of it affecting me in any way apart from my shyness, assumed that a person from such a background would surely be delinquent, uneducated or feral. It had come as a great surprise for them to learn that, despite my harsh early life, I had developed well in many aspects, including when it came to social etiquette, values and respect for others.

I continued to try and articulate this, but to no avail; as far as they were concerned, according to some of their textbook training, my unfortunate early years surely somehow made me doomed to not being able to manage in life. 'But I have never had any issues relating to any social or psychiatric matters. I mean, I am reserved in personality, but I have never had any issues of the mind; rather, I have something of a problem with my reproductive system, which no one will take seriously,' I tried to quietly plead.

But the junior psychiatrist exclaimed, 'But that is the very problem, in the sense of the mind, Rebecka! The pain and bleeding are psychosomatic; it is emotional pain from childhood, manifesting itself as physical pain.'

'But my experiences from my early life have never particularly troubled me to that extent,' I answered respectfully, 'you would never have even known about them if I had not been given that initial assessment, when I was in hospital for the gynae symptoms'.

As I sat, feeling perplexed, she continued, almost smirking, 'With this pain and bleeding that you think you have, what do you expect us to do? '

A feeling of humiliation crept in within me, at those words.

I simply answered, softly but sincerely, 'I did not ask to come here or to speak to any psychological health professional; I know my own mind. I do not want anything from the medical professionals other than help for my gynae symptoms. I would not waste the doctors' time if I did not genuinely have them. My background has never been a big deal to me—so why is it to you?'

'Because,' she answered, 'as we have explained, it is the reason why you are perceiving physical symptoms that are not real.'

She then asked me questions regarding my current living circumstances and even my diet. 'So, you're starving yourself,' she somehow concluded, upon my answering that I liked to eat healthily.

'No, please, I am not.' I softly replied. 'Why do you think this?'

'Because you have a BMI measurement that is lower than average,' she answered.

'My BMI is at the lower end of the scale, that's all; it's still healthy. My weight is in the normal range, especially for being athletic as a dancer. Please may I ask, why does that matter so much?'

She did not answer but instead asked, 'Does it make you feel like you have some control over your life to be slender? You had no control over your life when you were a child, so do you feel that maintaining slimness now gives you some control?'

I politely answered gently, 'Well, that is nonsensical, isn't it? No person has any control over their life as a child, so why should I be bothered if I didn't either? I'm simply slim because I have been athletic for all of my life and I make healthy choices with what I eat.'

I empathise with those who genuinely have problems with certain issues—but in my personal case, I knew myself and my own behaviour very well, and these issues and questions surrounding them were not applicable to my life in any way.

The junior psychiatrist continued with her questioning. 'Do you self-harm? Cut yourself?'

'No,' I quietly responded.

'Have you ever thought about cutting yourself?'

'Of course not, no.'

'I see you are wearing a long sleeved top,' she observed.

I was puzzled. In my usual tone of voice I politely added 'It's winter. I am wearing a sweater because of the cold weather.' I looked over at Ethan at this point and, sure enough, he returned my puzzled look.

'I expected you might be covering your arms,' the junior psychiatrist said, looking pleased with herself. She asked to see my forearms.

With embarrassment, I responded quietly, 'Gosh, this is so degrading' as I adjusted the sleeves of my sweater and held my arms, outstretched, in front of her, displaying my wrists.

She leaned in to have a good examination at the perfect, unflawed, unmarked complexion of my wrists and arms and seemed almost like she could not believe it, to have not found any evidence of self-harming, from the recent or far past.

There appeared to be no end to the searching for trying to find something wrong, however.

'Do you have strange thoughts?' she pressed on.

'No, I don't feel that I do.'

'Any suicidal thoughts?'

'Absolutely not, no,' I responded.

'And what about criminal behaviour?'

'Pardon?'

'Have you ever been in trouble with the police?' she asked, looking directly at me.

I was perplexed. 'No. I would never behave like that'.

'And what about addictions? Have you ever used drugs? Do you abuse alcohol?'

'No, none of those things.'

'None at all? Are you sure?' she asked, regarding me with utter surprise.

'Absolutely none at all', I replied politely, though with quiet frustration at now having to explain myself in this way, all for just asking if I could please have help with the pelvic pain issues. 'I've never had any of these things in my life.'

They could not understand that, contrary to some traditional thinking, given that I had been around so much abusiveness in a deprived depressing situation in my formative years, I was always drawn to the total opposite of my circumstances, that being the pleasant, civilised, interesting, healthy and bright things in life.

When I politely challenged their illogical theory, I was simply told, 'That's not possible, Rebecka. Our early years define who we are.'

If that truly is the case, then yes, my early years had defined me with shyness and, as I would later appreciate, my own poor boundaries which meant that I would be too tolerant of others mistreating me—but that aside, they had also defined me as a person who had consideration for others, was resilient and emotionally independent and wanted to live a peaceful and healthy life. Hence, as a person who believes that we can overcome awful experiences in our early lives so that they do not have to define us or rule our lives, and that it is entirely possible to go on to lead a balanced life as an adult, I found the psychiatrist's textbook broad statement of hopelessness regarding anyone from a background like mine utterly depressing.

But as usual, my lack of assertiveness with others and ever-present politeness meant that I was reluctant to stand up for myself, least not to medical professionals for whom, as a whole, I had immense respect. Instead, having tried to plead my case as graciously as possible, I remained completely quiet and kept my concerns inside; that was the way that I always dealt with everything.

Upon finishing her questioning and writing down my responses, Ethan began to speak. 'She doesn't have problems with her mind; I know that because I live with her, and I have also worked with mentally ill people. Her pain and bleeding symptoms are real. She should not have been referred here.'

'Well, the psychiatrist who assessed her in the hospital where she reported the gynaecological symptoms believes this referral to be correct on the basis of the cervical screening tests being normal, as well as his findings during the assessment; that is, her deprived and abusive early years and adolescence.'

'It seems, with all respect, that you are just looking for anything to attribute her physical symptoms to, despite her telling you repeatedly that she has no significant problems from her early life.'

'Her childhood experiences are manifesting themselves as perceived physical pain, just as we would expect from someone from her background,' the junior psychiatrist told Ethan.

I was so frustrated at where they had at arrived at that from. They had asked me routine questions on my background such as, 'Did you enjoy school?' and I answered nonchalantly, 'I loved the learning aspect, but was violently abused and beaten throughout my school years, so I couldn't wait to leave.' Then, they responded, 'Why were you beaten?' to which I shrugged, still in a composed manner, 'So I was repeatedly told, mainly because I was very poor, but also because I looked different, had a dancer's physique and a soft voice and was incredibly shy'. But I overcame my early life, and I have never let it hold me back.'

That was enough for the psychiatrist to seize on my background, even though I had succinctly stated that I had overcome it, and I was not having problems from my earlier experiences, apart from the practical aspects of my background making it virtually impossible to access the career in the arts that I had been selected for. Sure, my adolescent years had affected my self-esteem initially and formed me with a lack of assertiveness with others and this had perhaps held me back in some ways, but I was not distressed by them and had never suggested as such, either in my words or behaviour. My 'life is what you make it' attitude could not have been expressed any more clearly.

I had tried to give the benefit of the doubt initially, in my thinking that they had perhaps been well-meaning in their intentions, possibly thinking that they are helping me in some therapeutic way, simply because of learning of my early life. But it was very apparent that this was not the case, as they were not at all interested in how my adolescent years had actually affected me, in being reserved and not having strong enough boundaries, instead only expressing intrigue and at times, had an attitude vaguely pertaining to mockery.

'So there is nothing wrong with her mind? No diagnosis of anything to do with mental health?' Ethan gently enquired.

'There is no diagnosis at present,' answered the junior psychiatrist reluctantly.

Ethan added in a polite manner, 'So now that you can see that she does not have mental health issues, could you please consider the possibility that the physical symptoms are not psychological, but are actually real?'

Without giving this any thought, she retorted, 'Although she does not have mental illness, that does not mean that her insistence that she is experiencing pain and bleeding is not psychosomatic. This could be a trauma response to her earlier experiences. I am referring her for further assessment for depression and antidepressant medication.' She glanced at me before continuing, 'if she refuses this, we might have to take other measures'.

My stomach turned at hearing these words, as I quietly pleaded, 'Please. I really am having problems with pelvic pain and bleeding!'

But she ignored me. I was gripped with fear now, clasping a hand to my mouth in quiet angst. Ethan tried to politely intervene to put a stop to this ludicrous situation, but she dismissed his concerns with a flippant, 'It's good that you are supportive, but as we have explained, these physical symptoms are psychosomatic, based on her childhood experiences.'

'But she has been very open about her earlier years, and it has never affected her apart from her being shy sometimes!' Ethan gently insisted. 'She never complains about her early life at all or says that it bothers her.'

But the psychiatrist was insistent that my physical symptoms could not be possible. 'An appointment letter will be sent to you for further assessment,' she explained, 'and I will write to your doctor to recommend a prescription for antidepressants.'

And with that, we left, both of us bewildered. Ethan said sincerely, 'I am sorry, I didn't think it would be like that; I thought they would meet you and realise that they've made a mistake and retake the gynae tests. I didn't think you'd be so judged for your early life being the way it was. I don't know what to do.'

I never told anyone else at all about what I was going through—mainly out of total embarrassment at my strange predicament.

Meanwhile, the modelling feature for the newsgroup shoot was supposed to include an article detailing my interests and hopes for the future. For this article, I was asked if I had always wanted to be a model. 'No, I never thought about it. I was severely abused all through my teen years, partly for the way that I looked, so I never considered being a model, even after being invited to be one'. I answered. Would I give my support to young people going through similar experiences, I was asked? I had responded in the affirmative.

Despite the feature having not come into print, a couple of press feature writers from different agencies and publications had learned that I might be becoming something of a possible emerging talent after a difficult start in life and how I might possibly go on to achieve a bit of something within the arts or as a model, so they asked me to do a feature for them. These enquiries were not for anything major, and I expect that I was not at all of much interest to those making them, but they just seemed to think me to be a nice girl, who had overcome something and might go on to do some good things with whatever talent I was kindly deemed to have.

However, I had absolutely no interest in pursuing publicity; I explained that I only wanted to focus on developing professional, creative work, that being a little photographically but more interestingly, as a writer and performer, rather than the press features.

'Would you be willing to speak about the abuse that you suffered as a teenager?'

'If it will help anyone, then yes, I suppose so,' I responded nonchalantly. 'But I would rather that I am not defined by that. I want to put all of that behind me'.

'What did your abusers say to you?' they asked.

Though I tried to make light of the matter, I attempted to explain, without going into detail, that I was violently physically and emotionally abused throughout my adolescent years, for the combination of how I looked and spoke, being poor, a creative and incredibly shy.

But the reporter took the offhand comment I had made about my 'particular body shape' the wrong way. I therefore had to explain how my physique was always very slim and toned and that partly because of this I was selected to be a dancer and model.' That was the point, though I did not understand it at the time: apparently the perpetrators hated that, so they wanted to give me more of a complex about myself', I said. But they seemed to focus on that unimportant subject, and the way in which they wanted to present it was not either relevant or accurate.

They told me that they wanted to do a nice feature on the work that I might be beginning to establish, I asked a professional within modelling if this was okay. Their response was, 'It won't do any harm. It is not scandal, just a nice feature. They like you because you are a lovely appealing girl who may possibly have a chance of doing well for herself after overcoming a bad start. Just go with it.'

A friendly media guy told me. 'You look great; but putting that aside, I think there is more to you than that. Readers like young women with the qualities that you have, especially if you have the talent to go with it.'

Despite his kindness and compliments, however, he wanted me to discuss family and where I lived but I didn't want to make mention of that at all.

I began to fear that I might never escape others defining me by the deprived and abused circumstances of my early life. *Why is that so important to them when it isn't to me?* I wondered. I only ever wanted to focus on where I might be going in life and not be pulled back by my unfortunate start.

In a nutshell, I did not feel comfortable with what the couple of feature writers were asking of me, as they wanted to say that I liked things that I, in fact, disliked or had absolutely no interest in, in order to promote whatever the interests of a certain publication might be.

It all felt rather ridiculous, and I decided that I did not want to do the features.

Later, one of the features writers who contacted me who I *did* feel comfortable possibly agreeing to do something of a light-hearted feature with, however, was a friendly woman in her thirties and had some sensible ideas for nice pieces that she wished for me to work on. She had no interest in where I came from; only in what I might do in the future. Hence, I agreed to chat to her.

'Would you do an interview with me? I would like to offer it to the high-end women's magazines,' she said excitedly. 'We think good things are going to happen for you; the guys in the office are *besotted* with your photos! You could go far in life, but you will be liked just for being who you are. You're a star in the making, and *we* can see it!'

But I dismissed these incredibly generous words merely as comical hyperbole; I was not convinced that anyone would be interested in me to that magnitude.

I explained my reservations to the nice reporter and told her of my not feeling good enough to be in the media. I had not achieved anything great so far, and therefore, as far as I was concerned, had no place or reason in being there; I felt that if I might go on to create something that, if I was fortunate enough, might become well-received by audiences or readers in the future, then in that case, I would feel there was at least some sense in participating in a media article for that work, if those audiences or readers wanted me to, but for now, I had not achieved anything like that.

'Oh, you'll overcome it with experience in the business,' she reassured me.

She was sensible about my very fledgling work within the professional world that I was entering and thought that it might be helpful to me to make a nice feature out of it. I still wasn't sure if I was good enough for this but agreed to speak with her further as she was kind and really friendly.

At this time, I was still preoccupied with the knowledge that I had to bizarrely, go for a further psychological assessment in order to hopefully receive assistance for the physical symptoms, and having that looming over me was not only bewildering but acutely embarrassing. I was also still dealing with the ongoing painful symptoms. Thus, whilst I wanted to progress with my prospective career, I could not tell the reporter about any of what I was going through.

Nonetheless, she was very pleasant to me and not demanding in the slightest.

'I think you're going to do so well at anything that you try your hand at in the arts or entertainment!' she said to me. It was kind of her to say so, but I still could not comprehend any interest in me.

At the end of our chat, she seemed happy and excited with the prospective feature and what she could put together from it and would be putting it forward to the high-end magazines. Though wary about the prospect of this, especially as I thought that I might not be wanted in the public eye, I began to accept it as, like I had been advised, just something that occasionally forms a part of working within the industries that I was becoming part of.

In the meantime, I received another appointment with the psychology department.

'I do not want to go to these appointments. I don't need them,' I politely but desperately pleaded with my doctor. 'Please, why will nobody listen to me when I say that I am experiencing a physical health problem?'

'You are under their care now,' he replied unsympathetically. 'There is nothing more I can do.'

I told my doctor that I would be refusing the antidepressants that they offered, as although I certainly felt low due to my situation, I did not have a depressive illness; rather, it was treatment for the gynae symptoms that I needed, not antidepressants. But then I was chillingly told by one of the medical professionals, 'If you don't accept this voluntarily, then we may need to take steps so that you have to, as your psychosomatic symptoms could be due to depression.'

A feeling of terror flashed through me at these words, and I softly pleaded, 'I implore you, please, this is completely unnecessary. Please, don't do this to me.'

'We might have no choice if you keep insisting that you are experiencing pain and bleeding that does not exist,' they replied.

I was left frightened at their words, but Ethan assured me, 'they can't do that to someone like you, a girl who looks after herself so well and behaves nicely and is respectful of other people. That kind of action is for people who are mentally ill or a danger to themselves or others, which you absolutely are not', he replied reassuringly.

Elsewhere in my life, I continued to unwittingly attract attention, especially where I lived.

I was never under any illusion that the staring and comments I often received were for anything other than my simply being perhaps a little different to most around me. Though I did not have self-loathing, I did not think myself to be anything outstanding, especially as I had internalised those aggressive derogatory comments that women and girls where I had come from had told me about the way that I looked. It felt peculiar therefore that I was often of so much interest to others; to me, it was just the way that I was, and therefore I could not understand what the fuss was about. I considered myself to be just a normal person.

In some places, I am sure that nobody would have batted an eyelid at seeing me and I would be uninteresting to them, but here, people would stop me in shop queues and ask if they could touch my hair. 'I can't believe it's real,' they would often say, along with funny comments such as, 'You look like a doll!.' 'You have hair like a mermaid!'.

I was always courteous in return as this type of interest was kind and one that was coming from a well-meaning place of course rather than its alternative: some of those I came into contact with were not as kind in their reactions at the sight of me. I was often met with an aggressive random 'who do you think you are?' (we can only wonder what that essentially means). I would walk past these loud people with my head bowed, avoiding eye contact, so as not to have to endure them shouting at me in public.

Upon witnessing the aggression and abusive comments

directed at me, a kind lady, who told me that she had worked in fashion in London during her youth and was complimentary about my appearance and demeanour, adding 'People around here wouldn't know a model if they fell over one. But don't stop being your lovely self just to please them,' (though I was, of course, not of any significance whatsoever in modelling, far from it).

But I could do nothing about the way that I naturally was and had to continue to face the abusive comments, as I was still aggressively questioned to the effect of, 'What right do you think you have to dress/speak/look like that?' It was a very strange situation, especially when I avoided attention at all costs, so as not to have to deal with the anger of others.

I always had a feeling of not fitting in, never more so than where I came from.

The junior psychiatrist insisted that I attend again for a follow-up at the depressing building, as despite them not finding anything wrong with my mind, they still felt that my gynaecological symptoms were non-existent and, now after learning of the somewhat cruel manner in which I had been treated during my adolescence, wished to probe into this further. I absolutely did not want to go but was afraid of the consequences if I refused to attend. This time, I let Ethan speak for me.

He gently asked the junior psychiatrist why I had been told that I could be forced into further psychological analyses if I continued to believe the pain and bleeding symptoms to be an issue.

'Well, we have the right to enforce this due to her continuing reporting physical symptoms that clearly do not exist, as the tests have shown and this might be due to depression as a result of her early years', responded the psychiatrist.

Ethan had experience of working with people who have mental illness, so therefore, having concluded that I was not experiencing any issues in that regard, politely tried to state my case in a gentle manner, 'You can't legally do that, especially as there is no reason in her behaviour to. Why would you want to do that to someone who is mentally healthy?'

After a slightly pause, she replied, 'I agree with the hospital psychiatrist's original assessment: that Rebecka is manifesting childhood trauma that she is not aware of in the form of perceived physical symptoms of pain and bleeding. Her insistence on physical symptoms that do not exist is clear evidence of this'

I must have seemed visibly worried about where this was all heading, as Ethan spoke up for me in a gentle manner. 'But she hasn't shown any signs of childhood trauma whatsoever and has never said that anything from her early life troubles her, to you or the psychiatrist or anyone else. This was only ever meant to be a process of elimination so that you could see that her physical symptoms are actually genuine, but you seem to have turned this into something else.'

These assessments were deeply humiliating for me and not at all how I wanted to be living my young life, and all the while, I hoped that one of the medical professionals would spot that I genuinely had physical health problems. None of these assessments found there to be anything abnormal with my mind, and yet the psychiatrist and some of their colleagues were importunate in their theory of my gynae symptoms being 'trauma manifesting itself as perceived physical pain', attributing this to possible depression.

It never seemed to occur to those concluding this that distinctly, apart from the very specific symptoms of gynaecological pain and bleeding, I otherwise had no problems with my health either mentally or physically, nor had I complained of any. That should have at least provided a clue that the symptoms were in fact genuine.

Throughout this process of analyses, they would revert back to my adolescent years and the severe abuse that I had suffered, despite my saying that I had overcome it.

'So, you see, that is why you have these feelings of pain and bleeding: they are feelings from childhood experiences.' All very Freudian and theoretical—and, of course, completely inaccurate (I wonder why so much is placed on such out-of-touch-with-reality hypothesis and, to say the least, peculiar ideas, in certain areas of study of the mind, when there are far more sensible and balanced works concerning the mind that should surely be the more valued and implemented, such as those of *Maslow*). No matter what answers

I gave, they kept coming back to this, progressing to asking me questions about self-harm and eating disorders. 'This is what we would expect from someone of your early life,' they said, despite there being absolutely no sign of either ever in my life to prompt them to think this.

Strangely, they would insist on weighing me and continue to check my arms for signs of self-abuse, but they never found any: doing something like that would be unthinkable for me personally. In great embarrassment I softly asked, 'Why do I have to do this when I don't have any issues at all of this nature? It is so humiliating,' but the answer was always the same: 'Because of your early life, we have to look for these things to see how it might have affected you. It is procedure.'

I loathed being made to go through these embarrassing, unnecessary processes, but, afraid of what would happen if I refused, I felt I had no choice but to go along with them, enduring the painful pelvic symptoms that I was being refused medical care for all the while.

Though I was a mentally strong girl, because of my reserved nature, this simply was not being seen. 'What are you going to do Rebecka? Hmm?' a psychiatrist asked me. 'Are you going to keep thinking that you have this pelvic pain for the rest of your life?'.

They believed that if I repeatedly analysed my early life experiences, despite my already having overcome them, that I would somehow miraculously cease thinking that I had the gynaecological pain and bleeding symptoms.

The more I was not believed, the more my voice faded. Being humiliated or not being given the chance to explain (which was almost always the case throughout my life) when I politely tried to communicate something important, sometimes resulted in me sort of 'losing' my voice; I would simply become quieter until silent.

The confidence I had built up since my teenage years was being gradually torn down. In their ignorance of my true situation, these health professionals made me feel that I was apparently destined to be, as the product of a penurious, abusive background, terribly badly or unhealthily behaved in some way, despite there being absolutely no signs of this; to the contrary, I had been kindly noted from a young age, in one way or another, for my abilities and had been managing my life okay, considering the circumstances. I began to worry: *Am I normal? What am I doing that is wrong?*

'One of the psychologists must surely eventually see that your physical symptoms are real,' Ethan said. 'Then, the doctors might take the gynae tests again, or something.'

We both quietly despaired at the situation.

Whilst in this state of limbo, the nice journalist from the press agency called me again, wanting my permission to print the uplifting-style article in the magazines. However, by this stage, I had now lost all confidence in myself as a result of being subjected to degrading psychological assessments that I did not need, in which my pain and bleeding were completely written off as being all in the mind. I was suffering more and more from the gynaecological symptoms but was receiving no medical treatment for them. Instead, I was told (extremely wrongly, as it turned out), as is believed, seemingly without exception in some traditional parts of psychiatry, that my deprived and harsh start in life forever destined me to be defined by that, hence why they had labelled the pain and bleeding as imaginary.

Consequently, in such bizarre and deeply embarrassing and deprived circumstances, I could not find the confidence to face being in the media features that I was asked to do as a by-product of a bit of modelling or my prospective creative works as a writer.

'My apologies,' I told the nice journalist sincerely, 'but I cannot do the feature.'

She seemed very disappointed. 'Please do it Rebecka. It'll be really great for you. There's nothing to worry about with the feature. We've been talking about it in the office; about how the readers will adore you.'

'I'm sorry, but I really can't', I told the nice journalist. Things have changed; nobody will be interested in me. I haven't achieved anything yet. But thank you for being so nice.'

'But Beck, it would be *such* a shame not to do it,' the journalist insisted. 'Some of the magazines are interested in the feature.' She seemed really let down. Looking back, I can see why: she had gone out of her way being accommodating to me and we had gotten along almost as well as old friends do and her intentions were, indeed, to produce a genuinely nice feature. But I had begun to believe what the psychiatrist had (wrongly) inferred: that my being from a deprived and severely abusive background might make me, according to hypothesis, unacceptable, regardless of how healthy my mindset was, whatever qualities I was kindly deemed to have, or who I was as a person.

The journalist never got to know what had really caused me to feel the way that I did about myself and not feeling good enough at the time for the public or media aspects of working within modelling or the arts, and there is no way that I would ever have told her, no matter how likeable she was: I felt sheer embarrassment at my strange circumstances and thought that I would not be believed by anyone in any case.

Although I received occasional phone calls and enquiries of this nature from a couple of features writers over the next few months and though it was explained to me that press matters are sometimes part of modelling and the performing arts, I completely lost the confidence, because of what was going on in my life, to have anything to do with that part of things back then, and, quickly, the media people, in turn, lost their bit of interest in me.

I desperately wanted the unnecessary psychological evaluation to stop and to not have to see these people anymore, but it was not that simple: every time I went to seek medical help for the pain and bleeding symptoms, I was referred straight to psychiatry or psychology instead for the symptoms apparently being 'psychosomatic' or due to 'possible depression', despite there being no other reason at all to send me there. It was a vicious cycle that I could not get out of.

As a result, my self-belief in the manuscript that I had worked on—a book to help other young people to successfully get through tough times—had disappeared. I put the manuscript through the shredder, along with the basis of the novel that I had written—an action that I would many years later come to regret (especially as in the decades to come, similar styles and topics to what I had written would become popular). *Am I just fooling myself into thinking that I can ever achieve anything or be taken seriously with my creative work?*

I thought, *can someone from my background really do anything in this regard?*

The pain and bleeding, meanwhile, had not subsided, and had gradually and subtly worsened.

I found myself temporarily incapacitated at times with the intensity of this and would have to lie down with my knees almost to my chest or embracing a cushion to my abdomen. I was self-medicating the near-constant dull ache in my lower pelvic area that alternated with occasional sharp pains, with over-the-counter pain medication. I was not in agony (as I would discover later, this pain had nothing on that resulting from extensive radical surgery), but the pain was certainly disrupting my life, and the bleeding was frequent. However, as I always did in life, I told myself that I had to get through it.

Neither Ethan nor I could ever have imagined that anything as serious as a tumour could be present. After all, the cervical screening test had specifically ruled that out. Some kind of chronic gynaecological problem—polycystic ovaries or something similar—most probably, is what we thought, as we knew that there was something wrong in that respect.

Regardless, the psychological health assessments continued against my wishes.

'Please', I softly pleaded in deep embarrassment and confusion on one of these degrading occasions, in desperation for these analyses to end, 'I try to do my best in life. I respect others. I completely look after my health in every way. I don't know why I need these appointments.'

But the answer that I was always provided with remained along the same lines of 'the cervical screening tests have shown that you do not have any illness, so because we have established that you are from an abusive and poverty-stricken background, we know that the pain and bleeding that you have reported is psychosomatic as a result of possible depression due to the effects of your early years'.

By no means were all of the medical professionals involved in my care at the time incompetent or treated me badly, however, and some were really kind to me. At an appointment at psychology health services when it was being attempted to determine if my gynaecological symptoms were all in the mind, I saw a new therapist, who turned out to be an immensely affable guy in his late thirties. He asked some of the usual analytical queries but mainly questions that none of the medical professionals had asked me before. As usual, when asked about my adolescent years and the strange and rather brutal experiences that I was repeatedly subjected to, I was completely open in saying how they had left me with some shyness and self-doubt, but I had resolved early on not to dwell on it and to move on from it. He was pragmatic as I gave my answers, and he enquired about my interests, which he seemed to like chatting to me about. His care and concern shone through.

The psychotherapist asked me about how the gynaecological symptoms were affecting me and seemed sad and slightly emotional when I told him of them and how nobody would take them seriously. 'What strikes me,' he said, 'is that there is no history whatsoever of any issue of the mind before you were referred here, when you started reporting the gynae symptoms. The psychological assessments also do not show anything of concern at all.' He turned to look at Ethan with a puzzled expression. 'I don't understand why she has been sent to psychology or psychiatry services.'

'I don't either,' Ethan responded softly. 'They don't believe that she's really suffering from the symptoms; they think it's all in her mind, when it's not; emotional pain from childhood that she is not aware of, manifesting itself as imagined physical pain, they said.'

The psychotherapist looked deep in thought, and, reading through my medical notes, responded, 'Yes, I see from the notes that this is the assumption, but an assertion can't be made just on that one thing, and although they have assessed her extensively and talked about all aspects of her life with both of you, there has been nothing else noted about her other than that she looks a bit anxious and slim'. He paused and looked intensely thoughtful as he continued to address Ethan, '*I* would say that she's been very successful in overcoming her early life.' He turned to my direction, 'I believe you, Rebecka,' said the therapist reassuringly, 'and I think it would be expected that you would look a little anxious if you have pain that is not being treated—and I don't suppose it helps being sent to the wrong places! But I have to address your weight, as you have been referred here partly with a suspected eating disorder. Do you feel that you struggle with eating and your weight?'

Calmly and politely, I answered, 'No, I really don't. After the psychiatrist questioned me in hospital about my gynae symptoms and then my childhood, he stated that I looked thin. My BMI is on the lower end of the scale, but it is definitely not under-weight,' I explained. 'I have effectively been athletic for years, with my dance training and running and cycling everywhere. Also, for modelling and dance, I have to be slim. I eat healthily and exercise, that's all. I have none of the physical traits of an eating disorder: anyone who understands eating disorders can see this from the excellent condition of my hair and teeth. I've tried to explain this to the psychiatrist when questioned about it, but they won't accept my answer; to them, it can't possibly be that I'm just healthily slim and athletic.'

'Well, that makes sense to me,' the psychotherapist answered. 'Perhaps you need to slightly build up your nutrition, though, if you're experiencing blood loss; that can result in depleted nutrients—particularly iron. You may just need supplements to help with that, so just to be on the safe side, a nutritionist can help—but I can't find any reason to suspect an eating disorder. In fact, like in your other assessments, I cannot find anything particularly of note at all. I think you need your physical health assessing again; if you have an underlying physical condition that is not being treated, then that could make you feel a bit low. I will refer you to the nutritionist for the reasons I have discussed. It's difficult, as your gynaecological screening tests results have been noted as normal, but you are clearly experiencing pain. I wonder if a second opinion from a gynaecological consultant, or perhaps retaking the tests, would be helpful?' he mused. 'I can suggest that it might be appropriate for your pain and bleeding symptoms to be investigated further, if possible. Obviously, I am not a specialist of physical health, but I can try to get you referred to those who are.'

This wise psychotherapist had the intuition to understand that I was genuinely suffering from physical symptoms.

Addressing both Ethan and I, he continued, 'I will try my best to see if I can recommend a referral to the gynaecology department through your doctor. I know that you have been there before, but perhaps further testing could be done. I am not an expert on physical health, but I think that I should definitely discuss with your doctor how we can help you.' He paused. 'I will see you again in around three months' time, just so that I can check you have been referred to the right place and that your physical symptoms are being addressed by the right departments before I refer you from our services back to those for physical health.'

The doctor shook my hand, and I thanked him sincerely, almost tearfully, with relief for actually being understood.

The expression on his face was one of real and profound empathy.

Finally, someone had actually seen me and treated me as a normal functioning girl —not a patient number from deprived and abusive beginnings who may be useful as a case study to try and (fruitlessly) prove Freudian theory about what someone from that background should become; but, in fact, a capable and pleasant young person who was suffering and, until now, had not been heard.

4
Never-Ending Torment

A MEDICAL STORY THIS IS not.

But, it should be said that whilst the health service changed my life forever for the worst, separately, it also saved that very life, and I would not be here today without the goodness and skill of some of the brilliant specialists, doctors, nurses and anaesthetists whom I would later go on to be under the care of.

Whilst 'I am just doing my job' is what many of them modestly say, there is a distinct difference between doing that job with ethics, care, and competence—which the majority of medical professionals certainly do—and then the opposite of that, which fortunately is rare but seemed to have featured in my experiences of some of the medical care that I received.

Such worrying experiences began with my reporting the symptoms of the gynaecological pain and bleeding.

I had now been suffering from the pain and bleeding for around three years. What had begun as an only slightly noticeable difference, slowly increased in severity over the years.

A few months after meeting with the wise psychotherapist who had realised that I had been wrongly referred for psychological care, an appointment letter arrived for the unpleasant psychology health services clinic.

I was, however, not too worried this time: I knew I would be seeing the trustworthy male psychotherapist that I had spoken to previously, and thus knew it would be the last time I would ever have to go there, as a medical professional had now accepted that my symptoms were genuinely physical, and I had no need to be seen at this department

Ethan and I went there, believing that this would be the last time I would have to attend any of these types of places—but when we were led into the consulting room, we were instead met with the smug junior psychiatrist, who informed Ethan and I that the psychotherapist had been transferred to another department.

'He said that I didn't need to be here', I quietly explained, 'he was going to help refer me for further tests for the pain and bleeding,'

But she responded, 'He wrote to your doctor and requested a retaking of the tests you have already had done, but the doctor refused to do so due to the fact that you had already been tested for everything. The psychotherapist's opinion is not the same as mine and the psychiatrist who saw you in hospital (on the gynaecology ward). As we have said, you require further psychological assessment due to your insistence that you have gynaecological symptoms which have been proven to not exist and which we think are because of your neglected and abusive early years which might indicate possible depression.'

I was distraught at these words and became tearful with fear and frustration.

Ethan politely but firmly asked, 'But what about the blood test results showing some abnormalities?'

'Your doctor has said that the result differences are slight and could be caused by no more than a common cold. It is Rebecka's reporting of gynaecological symptoms that clearly do not exist that is of concern; the behaviour in this regard is consistent with that which we would expect for someone from her background'.

Ethan politely queried. 'Can I please ask what behaviour? Her pain and bleeding? Her shyness? This does not seem right to be so judged on her early years for having been poor and abused, especially as there had never been any problems from that before. She really is in *physical* pain'.

Ethan had tried repeatedly to get the correct medical help for me—for physical health—but almost none of the medical professionals would take his comments seriously, since as far as they were concerned, the tests had ruled out any physical issue.

After being humiliatingly analysed for anorexia and bulimia and finding that there was no evidence whatsoever for this, they dropped that theory and did not mention it again but instead increased the intensity of their focus on my early years, continually looking for reasons why I would have 'psychosomatic gynaecological symptoms' and continued to ask me questions regarding this.

'So when you feel the pain and bleeding, what abuse from your childhood do you remember?' There was no connection obviously, but it was insisted that there must be.

This again made me feel that I was somehow defective simply because of the misfortune of my beginnings, even though I had done my very best to overcome them. I hardly dared say anything to the medical professionals about this at the time; I believed that I had to do as I was told and be polite, perhaps because of the extreme respect for authority that had been instilled in me, and so this cycle of analyses continued.

By this point, most areas of my life had begun to be disrupted by the pelvic pain symptoms, including socially and with consistent work.

As much as Ethan and I both knew the symptoms to be there, neither him nor I thought them to be anything serious: chronic, disruptive, and painful, yes; but life-threatening and life-changing, no. All of the tests had certainly ruled that out.

Dismayed, Ethan very politely explained to the doctor how badly this situation was affecting my life. He had some medical training and experience that was sufficient in allowing him to understand the behaviour of the mind and body in these circumstances and he therefore hoped that the doctor would take into consideration his point of view that I was experiencing actual physical pain.

'It's good that you are being helpful and supportive, but you have to understand that the symptoms that she says she is experiencing are all in her mind,' was the doctor's response.

'With all due respect, they are not,' Ethan insisted. 'The pain and bleeding that she has is very real and is frequent. Something isn't right, physically.'

'Let me assure you, it is *not* physical; the tests have proven this. According to the psychiatric reports, she is interpreting emotional pain as physical pain,' replied the doctor.

By now, Ethan had heard quite enough of this consistent mono-logue between some of the medical professionals involved, and so he politely pressed on. 'I have experience in working with mentally ill people, and she does not have psychological issues; this is *not* in her mind. But by being subjected to psychological assessments that she doesn't need which you refer her for, you are actually causing her to suffer. She needs treatment for the physical symptoms, not for her mind.'

'Any gynaecological issues that she is worried about are just nor-mal female problems,' dismissed the doctor.

'Please, they're *really* not,' insisted Ethan. 'I am not a doctor, but from my experience as a medic, I understand them enough to know that she has genuine gynae pain and bleeding symptoms that she is not being treated for.'

The doctor was incredulous. 'Look,' he said, raising his voice slightly as he slid a file of test results and assessment notes towards Ethan, 'there is *nothing* wrong with her physically! The tests do not lie! All of the tests show that her gynaecologic health is fine, and the psychiatrists who have been asked to establish if her symptoms are psychological agree that it is the difficulties that she experienced during her childhood that are making her think she has a gynaeco-logical condition. As they explained, she is interpreting emotional pain as physical pain.'

Ethan politely questioned, 'If you don't mind me asking; why is it, then, that she has always been classed as completely healthy psy-chologically until the pain and bleeding started? That's still what she is classed as now; apart from them saying that she could possibly be a bit depressed—which she would be if she was not being listened to about her physical health. I understand that you are only seeing the test results as normal, but perhaps they need to be retaken. I have the greatest of respect for the medical profession, and we would never be timewasters of it—but *please* consider the possibility that *someone* has got *something* wrong in her diagnosis.'

At this point, the doctor seemed unable to contain his annoy-ance, and snapped, 'There are *no more* tests for her to have for these symptoms that she is imagining! It is agreed that it is *psychosomatic*!

If you don't like what you are being told, you can seek another opinion, but it is highly unlikely to be any different from what has already been determined.'

Ethan and I could both see that any further pressing of the issue, however polite and subtle we were about it, would be pointless. A second opinion was granted however, and the doctor who provided this was slightly more helpful, but again, he was blindsided by the negative test results. He reassured Ethan, 'Lots of young women have irregularities with their cycle, which often settle down by the time they have children. I would not say it is all in her mind; I cannot see that she has any kind of problem mentally, but that is just my opinion and is really for a psychiatrist to determine. I believe that she is just experiencing common fluctuations with her cycle, which can seem like irregular bleeding. The pains she is experiencing are normal cramps, which are worse for some.' He concluded, 'Whilst she is experiencing discomfort, she does not have a serious health problem; the tests would have picked it up if she had, and she is too young to have any kind of serious gynaecological problem anyway. So, there is nothing at all to worry about.'

'In that case, could you please give her any treatment at all for the pain and bleeding? It's seriously beginning to take over her life,' pleaded Ethan.

'We recommend taking over-the-counter pain relief and using a heat compress,' offered the doctor. 'It's just normal cycle fluctuations; please do not worry.'

I returned to see my doctor once more with the same symptoms, but he simply said, 'As I said it would be, the second opinion would not be much different. The tests prove that there is nothing wrong with you physically.'

'But—' I began to pleadingly reply.

'Rebecka,' the doctor interrupted, raising his voice in a now irritated manner, 'if you persist in trying to seek medical help for pain and bleeding, I will have to report it to psychiatry. We have established that you don't have pain and bleeding and that these symptoms that you are reporting are psychosomatic, so if they feel it necessary to involuntarily treat you for that, then they may be able to. There is nothing more that can be done.'

With these words, I was left bound by a mixture of intense fear along with frustration, and embarrassment. I had tried to politely plead for some help for the pain and bleeding symptoms but that was all I could do; answering back to a doctor would be almost unthinkable for me as that would be impolite and disrespectful, I thought. Therefore, I felt that I had to accept what the doctor told me, even though I knew so well that I had genuine physical pain. But really, I was also frightened of being forced into further analyses if I continued to mention the symptoms.

The physical symptoms became slowly increasingly troublesome, and Ethan became more concerned at how abnormal this was. I was admitted to the hospital with the symptoms three more times over the years, but they were never properly looked into, due to having already been stated as 'psychosomatic'.

The medical professionals tried to figure out where to place me, as due to the lack of any actual diagnosis, I did not fit anywhere, adding to the strangeness of the degrading circumstances that I sometimes found myself in.

I was unaware until much later that my particular and youthful appearance and reserved nature, combined with the circumstances that had been beyond my control made me especially vulnerable to abuses. On three distinct separate occasions during these years, I was subject to humiliating behaviour within a medical setting. Though I was not treated violently at such times, these incidences, I later discovered, would have been classed as violation. I would like to spare my dignity by not going into the details of them but suffice to say that I was handled and touched inappropriately, and at the time, I was afraid and too respectful of authority to say anything about it.

I accepted these incidences as simply yet another few degrading moments in the life that I never seemed to be able to protect myself within, no matter how optimistic, resilient and logically-minded I was; I often found myself in circumstances that those so inclined were free to take advantage of – and I never seemed to be able to do much about it.

These perpetually helpless circumstances, in almost all areas of my life at the time and my inability to get myself out of them, made me feel so absolutely mortified.

Thankfully, on a couple of occasions when admitted to hospital with the painful pelvic symptoms, I was under the care of some extremely nice doctors, who told me that they believed that I was physically suffering, but that, given the gynaecological testing had shown as normal, they were baffled as to what could be causing me pain. There are so many truly excellent doctors, and for me, being aware of that fact is how I balance out the bad things that occurred during my medical care.

Once, while in hospital. strangely, someone from psychiatry showed up to see me, citing the basis of them believing the gynaecological symptoms to be psychological and asking me the same questions they had in their previous analyses. The very empathetic young male doctor who was in charge of my care asked them psychiatrist why I was being psychologically evaluated, considering I had been admitted with physical symptoms, had no history of mental illness and was not displaying anything of concern in that regard. The psychiatrist took the doctor to one side and told him that he believed that the gynaecological symptoms were psychosomatic and due to depression—a notion that the doctor disagreed with, explaining how he was uncomfortable with a normally behaved, polite young woman being psycho-analysed against her wishes for the gynae symptoms she had been admitted to the hospital with.

A quiet debate ensued between the two clinicians before the psychiatrist left the ward with a steely expression and the doctor returned to my bedside, telling me that he would discharge me from the hospital for now. He then wrote to my doctor to raise the possibility that I should be re-referred to the gynaecological department for further testing. 'I think that we need to get the matter of the pain looked into further,' he said.

However, when a few months had passed and I still had not heard anything more about a re-referral to gynaecology, I asked my doctor about this—only to learn that the recommendations of the very conscientious caring doctor who had overseen my hospital stay had been overruled; it had been decided that no further investigation could be justified, since all the previous tests had ruled everything out.

Instead, and though I tried to refuse the appointments, I was referred for further psychological analyses. I called the relevant department to say that the use of their services was completely unnecessary, but, to my surprise, they returned by telling me that if I refused to attend, it would be reported to a psychiatrist who could seek action from my doctor for me to be given, effectively, treatment for delusions of gynaecological illness that they believed to be due to depression. Terrified that they would follow through with such action, I felt that I had no choice but to do as I was told, and so with great embarrassment, I attended the pointless meetings, one of which was, bewilderingly, for evaluation with a psychiatric nurse, despite my having no history of psychiatric problems or to be having any now. 'I don't need these appointments,' I gently told the kind and sympathetic woman. 'I just need help with the pelvic symptoms. As far as I am aware, I do not need help for my mind. But when I explain this, nobody will listen to me.'

'The doctors have confirmed that these are just normal female health issues. We can, however, feel heightened physical pain if we are in distress about something from our past', the nurse responded.

'I don't mean to be impolite, but I am not in distress about anything like that. I have never needed to talk about it at all,' I quietly explained. 'It has made me a reserved person, but apart from that, I learned to accept my earlier years long ago and I never dwell on them. It was the original psychiatrist who came to see me in hospital who brought the subject up, asking me general questions about it and then he seemed to make a big deal out of my background for no reason. It is the pelvic pain that I need help with, and nobody will believe me.'

As pleasant and empathetic as this lady was, I was by now exasperated at this continual response. It was clear that I was never going to be believed that my physical symptoms were genuine.

The psychiatric nurse asked me questions about myself, which led to my mentioning that I had been told by a psychiatrist that people from my neglected, abused and penurious background cannot achieve anything with their lives and that I would apparently therefore be destined to be some kind of nothingness. The nurse replied, 'Well, that's something I don't agree with. Just by speaking to you, it is completely apparent that there is no reason whatsoever for you to not be able to excel in life, especially with all your lovely qualities. You've got years left yet to pursue an opportunity to do well for yourself. I think you'll be absolutely fine with that.'

This did at least comfort me in terms of my now-shattered sense of self. Then, I told the nurse of how frightened I was at the suggestion that I had to continue with these analyses.

Sensing my quiet distress at this, Ethan politely said to the nurse, 'They are only allowed to do that to a person if they are a danger to themselves or others or diagnosed with some kind of mental illness—but it's been confirmed several times that none of those apply to her. She just needs further testing for the pain and bleeding she is experiencing.'

The nurse looked thoughtful as she responded to Ethan, 'Rebecka does not seem to me to have any mental or behavioural issues. But I do think she might be sad about something.'

Ethan politely replied, 'Well, if you don't mind me saying so, she is bound to be if she's in physical pain that is preventing her from getting on with her life. It might just be a small female health problem, but she still needs some kind of treatment for it,'

But the nurse, looking thoughtful, answered, 'The matter is out of my hands. I can give my opinion to the doctors, but it is ultimately their decision. I am powerless to intervene.'

The nurse explained that nothing could be done, as the psychiatrist's opinion seemed to count for everything. I despaired at how to get out of this situation and began to lose all hope that anyone was ever going to treat the mystery painful female health issue that I was increasingly experiencing. It seemed that the particular medical professional's original opinion—that the pain and bleeding must surely be all in my mind—had completely influenced the care of almost every medical professional who I saw, with the exception of the occasional doctor who tried to help me, having used their own intuition instead of placing all onus on generalised theory.

Having been declared stable-minded by the psychiatric nurse, the psychiatrist, rather than accept this, now tried different avenues of referral to psychology services, including referring me to see a cognitive behavioural therapist, with the objective seemingly being providing me with a sort of 'reframing' therapy that would allow me to see the pain for what it apparently, according to them, was: all in the mind.

Though I have nothing against certain forms of therapy, I was perplexed; *they think that they can fix the gynaecological symptoms by changing my behavioural patterns?*

I loathed having to once again face a humiliating analysis. *When will this end?* I quietly fretted, *what if I am trapped in this situation forever?*

The therapist was compassionate, friendly and softly spoken. But it turned out that she, too, would only listen to the psychiatrist's opinion based on the negative cervical testing results and having learned that I was from a very difficult start in life, and, as such, fully believed that my physical symptoms were psychosomatic. She asked me questions about my childhood and then about my frequent reporting of my gynae symptoms. 'So, you feel that you have pelvic pain and bleeding?'

I answered gently and with politeness, 'I actually *do* have pelvic pain and bleeding,'

She smiled warmly and looked sympathetic as she softly replied, 'Sometimes, Rebecka, when we are in unacknowledged emotional pain from our childhood, it can *feel* like we are in physical pain, and it can *feel* like we are bleeding, but we are not, you see.'

As ridiculous a statement as that was, this lady seemed a lovely person and I did not want to be impolite to her, so I simply quietly pleaded, 'Please, I implore you, I don't *feel* like this, I am *actually* experiencing these symptoms, and they are becoming worse. I am not in emotional pain; I am in physical pain.'

I could take no more of these degrading and unnecessary sessions that were destroying the confidence I had built-up since my adolescence, and I felt deeply embarrassed by them. Ethan could now see no point in them, either and he would help to get me out of this absurdity that was ruining my life. 'It's obvious they are never going to give you any treatment for your symptoms. I thought they would when they completely assessed you and found no mental illness, which should have ruled that side of things out, but this is ridiculous now. Just tell them you want these analyses to stop.'

But this proved not to be quite so simple. When I told those overseeing the appointments, that I would not be attending them anymore, they told me, "you can't do that. Once you are in this departments system, you are there for the rest of your life', (information that would later turn out to be wrong), which was news to me and which I found frightening. I should not even have been there at all in the first place. Desperate to get myself out of this degrading situation that I had never willingly entered but that had nonetheless allowed others to take control of my life with no valid reason, I knew that I had to stand up for myself.

It was difficult for me to do so because of my respect for medical professionals. But as it had been confirmed that I was of sound mind, I had no obligation or reason to be under any kind of medical care of this nature and so I politely explained this to the psychiatrist.

To this, they responded, 'You have to accept that our childhood defines who we are.'

The 'childhood' reference that had been so overused (given that seemingly everything in psychiatry is apparently related to childhood) was actually inaccurate; it had in fact been my *adolescent* years where I had been abused and most deprived, where I had been completely degraded for the way that I looked, my soft voice and shyness. However, I mostly overcame the effects of this by the age of twenty. But the questioning in the analyses would always come back to 'childhood'.

Anything I had achieved in my life, my qualities, and the way that I conducted my life and myself, was given little consideration: rather, the focus was totally on the theory that, according to some textbook areas of psychiatry, which are, as is often forgotten, only actually theoretical, my very unpleasant early life must have made me somehow incapable of being a fully functioning adult, despite never having shown any sign of this, apart from my diffidence.

But these are meant to be the professionals of the mind, after all, and so eventually, when they told me often enough that the pain and bleeding was all psychosomatic, I began to worry terribly that I might actually be defective in some way without my realising it. I had been classed as a completely normally developed young woman—so logic dictates that ultimately, such a worry is unfounded. But I did now feel thoroughly ashamed of being badly abused and living in penurious circumstances in my early life.

Occasionally, I softly tried to speak up for myself during these times, once answering the junior psychiatrist, 'The only problems that I have from my early experiences of being neglected and the emotional and physical abuse—and they *do* set me back, I openly admit—are reservedness and lack of assertiveness with others.'

'So, you see, you *are* affected by your childhood!' the psychiatrist exclaimed.

'Of course I am. Everyone is shaped to some degree by their formative and adolescent years. But in my case, this is in a small and *very* different way altogether to that which you imply, and it is not one that has ever required treatment for the mind.'

'Well, it is not, actually,' she quickly replied. 'You have psychosomatic pain and bleeding symptoms. This is exactly the type of behaviour that we would expect from someone of your background.'

It is stated in psychiatry that the formation of our earliest experiences affects the rest of our whole lives. This is the case in some way, as I do recognise that we all have a certain amount of 'programming' in us from our formative years—in my case, this definitely took the form of not protecting my own personal boundaries—but to define *everything* in this manner, especially in some of the traditional *Freudian* theories, and to assume that everyone reacts exactly the same way to the same experiences is, in my humble opinion, a conclusion without logic or fact.

I worried terribly about what I could do to get away from this absurd situation, and this preoccupied me greatly. None of this should have been happening to me and I should have been making a good life for myself, but now my sense of self and confidence had been almost destroyed as a result of me being repeatedly told that my deprived early life, including being violently beaten, would define me as apparently not being able to cope with life, no matter how normally functioning an adult I might be or how I very much so desired to press ahead with life regardless of its harsher experiences.

Eventually, I became quieter in my pleas to stop this cycle of unnecessary analysis, that was making me feel terribly embarrassed about myself. This reached a point where I practically said nothing at all to any of the medical professionals, because nobody (with the exception of that acutely intuitive psychotherapist) would listen to me.

But this situation became both frightening and depressing, leading to a rare moment of assertiveness with others borne out of the fear of knowing where my life would go if I allowed these people to continue to exert their professional power over it,

Ultimately, as Ethan had said, as I had not been found to have any mental illness and there had been no mention of anything pertaining as such up to the point of my reporting the pelvic pain, there was really nothing that could be done to stop me from requesting being referred back from the department where I had received the analyses: and I had to do it now, before they made this situation devastatingly worse.

Therefore, I proceeded to write a formal letter stating that I expressly wished to terminate these sessions at their department, outlining the reasons why.

Some weeks later, it was acknowledged that this action had officially been upheld. However, I was told, to my great angst, that now that a referral to such a department had been recorded, if I continued to report my pain and bleeding symptoms in the future, I would simply be referred back to the same place—and could even lead to me being forced into further psychoanalysis. Being told this filled me with so much fear that I would be very afraid to ever mention the pain and bleeding again to anyone, thus leading to me keeping it almost entirely to myself from then on, enclosing myself in a silent world of physical suffering.

Ethan and I resigned ourselves to the fact that I was not going to be treated for my gynaecological symptoms; rather, it was going to be something that I would just have to live with and manage as best as I could. I now knew all too well what could happen to me if I sought treatment for them again.

Although I received absolutely no treatment for the gynaecological symptoms in the end—indeed, the diagnosis of these was, at the time, entirely deemed to be psychosomatic—I felt a huge sense of freedom and relief that, after so much time spent allowing these professionals to analyse me in the initial hope that they would eventually see that my gynae symptoms were real, I was free from those who, in their arrogant certainty that their theory was correct, were continuing a downward spiral that could eventually destroy my life.

Happily, I had retained control of my own life—and I very much wanted to live it to the full. There were still possibilities for me to progress in the various aspects of my writing and performing, and I was prepared to work very hard for them.

But no matter how hard I tried to work my way out of my situation with determination and effort and by doing all of the right things, that would never be enough, as, although I didn't know it then, my circumstances were way beyond my control.

5
Struggling on Through the Bizarre

I TRIED AND TRIED TO plough on, placing all my effort into life, as is my natural way. However, all such efforts were ultimately in vain, as the painful physical symptoms of course continued.

This situation would go on for years; six more, to be exact, following the almost six years that I had by this time already been suffering with and reporting the pain and bleeding symptoms that would worsen slowly and subtly over time: never ceasing; taking over my life; consuming what should have been the best years of my life; sapping the life out of me (quite literally, as it would turn out).

The bleeding was, of course, never constant, but was frequent. The pain, however, gradually became a daily presence, fluctuating in its severity. Working and socialising was affected by this, and, as a result, I was prevented from living a normal young life.

My circumstances, however much I tried to get out of them and improve my life, always pulled me back and I often felt sad, worried and embarrassed because of them.

I tried to make it to bookings and castings when the symptoms were at their more tolerable and less uncomfortable, but this did not take away from the fact that I was struggling terribly.

Despite my pained state, I was still, surprisingly, continuing to sometimes unwittingly attract the attention that I had never learned how to deal with. It was not always horrible of course; people often openly paid me compliments. One of the loveliest of which I have received at times, from both sexes, is that they like my presence. I am not exactly sure essentially what it means or what they are sensing, but it is a great compliment to anyone when people spontaneously say that they feel truly good around you, just by being yourself. I have sensed this in others too, particularly in people who have no hidden agenda.

Compliments aside, there were also moments with the unexpected reactions which were outrightly peculiar.

One time, I was heading across London with Ethan to a commercial casting, wearing a dress, as I almost always do. Making my way through Leicester Square, I was a bit nervous to find a film premiere was underway and the area was busy, but we pressed on ahead. The stars of the red carpet seemed to have gone inside the venue. though the paparazzi were hanging around outside. For some reason, and goodness knows why, they noticed me. A couple of them did a double-take and readied their cameras momentarily. Ethan, who was accompanying me, began to laugh, as he said' they think you're someone famous, but they can't figure out who you are', and he chuckled at them as in their speculation, shouting over to each other, they tried to place me. I hurriedly tried to get past everyone in my embarrassment and felt ridiculous. But I could see the humour in this bizarre experience.

But whilst some experiences of being unexpectedly noticed in this way were amusing, others, however, were not.

On one occasion, I had been asked to perform as a dancer at a popular and stylish venue in Ibiza (the symptoms I suffered from had in that moment been under control enough for me to do so. With the pain and exhaustion from my physical symptoms, however, I almost collapsed immediately afterwards).

Well, one early evening there, I joined Ethan at a vibrant venue, frequented by celebrities but loved by all for the views.

On the way to the lavatories, I was stopped by a friend of the sportsman who was sitting in the VIP area with a group of people and with the sportsman staring intently at me. The friend asked me to join them. Politely making it clear that I had no interest in talking to any of them, I firmly declined their invitation and quickly hurried away and went into the loos.

There, some young women at the washbasins remembered me as a dancer from the nightclub earlier, telling me that they loved my dance style (a freestyle amalgamation of salsa and ballet that I had seemingly pulled off without anyone noticing that I had been in pain from the mystery symptoms) and were very kindly enthusiastic about my hair and appearance—all nice things, but as usual I found myself not knowing how to cope with being noticed. Regardless, I had no problem pleasantly chatting to others and they were absolutely lovely, so I obliged the conversations that some seemed to want to have with me.

At this point, the sportsman's partner walked in, accompanied by three of her friends, looking very stony-faced. Such women are often referred to in the media as WAGS (a term apparently meaning wives and girlfriends of sportsmen) but, in the politest sense, I was not interested in that world and so was indifferent to their presence and continued my conversation. However, they appeared to be staring directly at me. *That is odd,* I thought to myself. *Maybe I am just reading too much into it.*

They were listening intently to the conversation that I was having about dance with the lovely girls who wanted to chat to me, and I felt somewhat embarrassed that they seemed livid about people wanting to speak to me.

The atmosphere had changed from calm and happy to significantly tense and awkward when the WAG and her friends had walked in, and I felt uneasy about this and the fact that others seemed to be nervous around them.

I was stunned when it suddenly became clear that the sportsman's fiancée and her friends had not come to use the loos but had instead come to approach me. As I started to walk past them, they attempted to block my path as I made my way through the open doorway.

'Who are you?' demanded one of the friends, as they blocked the doorway to try and stop me leaving.

'Excuse me; may I get past?' I asked in a diplomatic, friendly way, ignoring their question.

They responded by mocking the way that I spoke by using a puerile exaggeratedly clipped cut-glass English accent: 'Oh, *excuse me, may I* get past...'

Ignoring their attempt at an intellectually challenging response,

I tentatively moved past the clique. But the WAG and her friends tried to get me to react, unleashing a tirade of loud verbal abuse.

Back outside, I could hear them shouting behind me, aggressive demeaning comments about my appearance, voice and the way that I walked

What on Earth was I doing wrong?, I wondered, assuming, as always, that the problem must surely be me.

I realised that they were following me as I re-joined Ethan, who had been oblivious to what was occurring—that is, until the angry group came marching up to us.

'What's wrong with *them*?' Ethan asked me, with a puzzled look.

'Well, I don't know much about them, but one of them is the partner of the sportsman in the VIP area,' I explained. 'One of his mates approached me and I said that I was not interested in being around them and was here with you. Those women came into the loos and got angry when the girls wanted to talk to me. They started shouting at me'.

Then suddenly our conversation was interrupted. 'Hair extensions!' bizarrely screamed the 'WAG' at me angrily (who, very oddly, unlike me, actually had them herself, which was confusing!).

Her friend quickly added to this by shrieking further insults about my appearance.

Silently, I stood in astonishment at this stunningly puerile behaviour, wondering what I had done to prompt it. I do not ever communicate on that level and refused to be drawn into it, instead not reacting and saying nothing at all.

Thankfully, they had followed me out of a side entrance, where I met up with Ethan and which did not lead onto the main area, where there were lots of people.

But I have always loathed public displays of this nature and find them to be crushingly uncomfortable. Ethan noticed that I was dissolving into discomfort as they continued to follow me.

'What is your problem?' he calmly, without raising his voice, challenged the WAG and her companions in response to their shrieking. 'Her hair isn't extensions, it's all her own; everything about her is natural.'

With that, the WAG, astonishingly, burst into tears and

continued to have some sort of meltdown, being comforted by her screeching friends, as Ethan and I quietly walked away.

'I think they were planning to corner you,' Ethan said as we paced away from the aggressive, screeching group.

'But I don't know what I've done wrong', I said, bemused.

'You did nothing wrong. You're just not anything like them.'

It was a strange experience, but I tried to bear in mind that many other women at the venue had been so friendly to me.

This bizarre encounter would unfortunately not be my only one of this type, as for some unfathomable reason, though I was not anything at all to do with their world, these women sometimes made an aggressive inquisitive beeline for me if I happened to be in any place that they were in.

On one occasion, at a trendy members-only London nightclub that I had been invited to by a showbusiness agent who wanted me to meet people in film and modelling who might want to work with me, there were different kinds of people there in the public eye, from various professional fields, but there were also some of the similar 'WAG' women, as I had previously encountered. I had walked into the place with an unassuming attitude as usual, thinking myself to be unimportant and was more than happy to let others shine. But though I was nothing at all to do with them in any way and hadn't spoken to anyone that they knew, when they saw that others were talking to me, they came over to me in a group, with an attitude of instant hostility.

When they established that I was merely a struggling, completely unknown fledgling voiceover artist, writer and dancer, doing a bit of modelling, completely devoid of any wealth or social status or connected to anybody, they cackled amongst themselves about how lowly they though that to be. They were ignorant to the fact that I had been offered their route to some kind of apparent status in life many times and deliberately and absolutely turned it down and stuck to my principles. Media profile and the social status of who someone's partner was, meant everything to them in a person. Qualities and strength of character in an individual meant nothing to their shallow minds.

Just as previously, my appearance, from what they told me, was once again an issue to them. It is a matter of personal choice what people wish to do with their look; I never interfere with what others choose to do in that regard, as it is simply none of my business, and I have no problem in accepting others regardless of if they have different interests or tastes to my own. For me personally however, I have never had any of the cosmetic procedures, extensions, fillers, and so forth.

But these particular women had, with no reason, a problem with that. That was their opinion, and I could handle it, but it baffled me as to why some seemed so compelled to tell me about it when there was nothing at all to prompt them to.

Their behaviour reminded me of some of those who I had previously been forced by circumstance to live amongst, who never seem to mature in their mentality. I did not respond at all—and I never would; not to any of them. I simply looked away while they continued cackling and thankfully my response made these types of unintelligible encounters very brief.

At other extremely fleeting moments in my life, I had met some nice women who were married to well-known sportsmen, so knew that not all were like that. But those in particular here were of a different ilk. There is no respectful or nicer way of telling it really; it was starkly apparent that trying to secure a famous man in order to be seen as top of the tree within their world was their main achievement in life, and what they felt to be important and were interested in was all terribly vacuous. That is their prerogative of course, but theirs was a world that I was entirely separate from and wanted absolutely nothing to do with and as such, I wondered why they had ever needed to bother me at all. It was a mystery that I decided not to waste any time on, however.

Along with this, there were other types of obnoxious unwanted attention too.

In this same place, I turned down the creepy advances of an acutely dull public figure, who seemed to be used to getting his own way. He was not happy about my outright refusal to get involved with him and caused a fuss, storming off in a mood with his companions trailing in his wake because he had tried to use his status to influence me into spending time with him and I had responded that besides not being single anyway, I was interested in what a person's character was like, rather than their status.

Earlier on that evening, I had found myself in the strange situation of being chatted to by a couple of paparazzi, who were hanging around outside the venue, presumably waiting to snap celebrities leaving the place in compromising situations. It seemed that the aim of their subtle questioning was for the press to get information about the famous people inside. 'You look gorgeous; who are you dating?' , one said to me.

Upon informing them that I was uninteresting to the press and was unconnected to anyone in the public eye, they soon left me alone, though they seemed to appreciate my humour.

'You should have let them take your photo. That's how to get known,' said a woman inside the nightclub, who worked in the modelling business.

'Well, I won't ever do that; it doesn't interest me whatsoever', I replied.

Another woman who was connected to showbusiness and whom I did not know was bemused, stating, 'But it's all about where to be seen and who to be seen with.'

'Not for me it isn't,' I responded, firmly, 'All that matters to me is doing some good quality creative work in the arts.'

I had come to learn of the behaviour of some who frequented these venues where celebrities were often present but were very dismissive of those of us in the arts or entertainment industry who were not famous, as they were instead only fixated in being attached to the media and celebrity world in order to promote themselves.

Their ruthlessness shocked me, but I kept my opinions very much to myself, as I was always aware that whatever others wanted to do was no concern of mine. Regardless, many an overambitious social climber would have fallen over themselves for the opportunities that were presented to me in this respect by particular men—and, indeed, some women simply could not understand why I would rebuff such offers. They thought me to be foolish and ridiculed me for entirely staying away from it all, but I never wavered in my stance.

Well, the adage of 'just because you can doesn't mean you

should' is one certainly worth keeping in mind.

I was still being told that I needed to attend some of the social occasions in the industry in order for me to be given work within it. I did not quite know whether that was the case or not. But though the effects of the mystery gynae symptoms meant that I was practically never socialising, on the couple of very rare occasion when I could manage to (and it was rare indeed), and had been able to earn the funds to travel into London for castings and auditions and so was there anyway, I would attend, as I hoped that at least these occasions might mean that I could meet other creatives and that we could perhaps even work on something together.

But I hardly ever seemed to meet the cool people; I would have liked to have chatted to the brilliant performers, filmmakers, technicians, sound engineers, actors and actresses, thinkers...all kinds of people within the arts and world of entertainment and also a few of those nicer people in modelling. However, through sheer bad luck and perhaps by way of my vulnerability, I rarely got the chance to, and more often than not, I only seemed to encounter people at these places or events who wanted to use me in some way, though at the time I was not fully aware of that. Later in life, it was explained to me that due to the combination of my qualities and vulnerability, I was attracting people with dishonourable intentions without my realising.

Further, I sometimes found that some would promise the world professionally, but would change completely in personality only hours later, for no apparent reason, or drop people like hot potatoes once the person was no longer considered useful to them. It certainly was not just me who was subject to this fickle disregard, as even some very established professionals within these fields have been treated badly in this respect.

There are many people in the world of the arts and entertainment, whether well-known or not, who are wonderful not just for the awesome talents that they are, but also as who they are as individuals, with their qualities and values—and it was those who I would have liked to converse with on these occasions. I wanted to be around the deep-thinking people who are caring with one another when they work together. But I never had the opportunity to meet them at this point in my life.

Instead, I often found myself amongst the unscrupulous attached to this arena, who usually seemed to almost surround me at such places.

On one occasion, I was introduced to a professional within film at the exclusive nightclub that I had been invited to, who seemed taken aback to meet me. He kissed my hand and, oddly, proceeded to talk to Ethan, not me, about my career prospects. He insisted that it would be better for my professional focus for me to travel alone overseas for work and attempted to reassure Ethan that I would be well looked after. But despite some of the other professionals assuring Ethan that I would be fine, he pleaded with me not to go anywhere with these people alone. Later, I would come to understand that I had at times been preyed on by some, but I did not fully realise it at the time (a couple of years earlier, a man who was a model agent had tried to persuade me to go abroad for modelling work. It was all very legitimate, with some well-established people, but Ethan had a bad feeling about that invitation too. In the end I decided not to go. Years later, it would transpire that by not going, my safety had been well and truly protected on such an occasion).

In this environment, on a couple of occasions, I also found that some could be under the influence of their 'powdered friend'. People who have been forced into the use of drugs I feel deeply sorry for, but those here were entirely different; they freely chose to partake in this and expressed that not only did they think it to be clever but also that they could not have cared less about how their actions might affect anyone else. But whatever they chose to do was absolutely nothing to do with me and so I said nothing at all and stayed away from their behaviour. They mocked me for never having tried drugs, but that did not bother me at all: I was steadfast in knowing that I would never touch them.

As if that was all not enough to try and navigate in this arena, encountering people who will do absolutely anything in the pursuit of fame is disconcerting indeed. Falling into fame as a by-product of success through brilliance in talent and dedication to working at something is one thing. Wanting to pursue fame as though it were a job in itself, is however, quite another. Well, some who were uninterested in true talent or values had tunnel vision regarding fame and their seeming intentions to misuse it. For Personally, with regards to this, I would rather be a 'nobody' with integrity, than a 'somebody' without it.

But I did not let it bother me too much. I wanted nothing at all to do with these types of goings-on and instead, I just wanted to focus on developing any artistry that I was kindly deemed to have, put the work in and be as consistent and dedicated as I could possibly manage (and I really did try to do so in spite of my circumstances). Although I myself was only on the very peripheries of this arena that connects with showbusiness, as some kind of a fledgling creative, and in my total insignificance as a completely unknown one, I hoped that that those thoroughly lovely people, at all levels of the arts and entertainment industry, might have felt this way too.

What I did really want to do within this professional world, was some engaging, meaningful creative work, and that was where my focus was.

Have you ever felt totally frustrated with your life? Perhaps you may have found yourself in a revolving door type situation that you feel you can never escape, no matter how hard you try?

Well, at this point, I now had two major issues in that respect: my background and its humble beginnings holding me back by way of lack of access to the avenues to the profession that had sort of selected me, and my health, in the sense of the gynaecological symptoms—and, no matter how much effort I placed into carrying on regardless of both, always refusing to let either be an excuse, this proved to be not so simple: both were now completely out of my control. I began to wonder whether these two elements would ever cease to be a hindrance to me.

A professional of the arts sternly advised, 'The problem is, you are not connected to anything relevant. There are many in the arts and modelling who don't have a famous parent or partner, but they have nearly always been to stage school, been part of a performing arts group at university or have a connection to a professional or an establishment in the arts or media. You haven't got that. Someone like you who has all the right requirements but who is unknown and has no connections at all can only do well in this if you get given a break for your talents; that's just the way it is.'

While a model agent told me, upon learning that I had been 'discovered', if you can call it that, as a bit of a model and creative a few years earlier, 'If you had done the features in the media then that would have launched your career. Without that you will really struggle as you have no media profile, you have no connections, and you are unknown'. But I could never tell them why such things had not worked out at the time and why I had felt that media things were not really for me, and nobody ever knew what I was going through; it was too embarrassing and strange to even attempt to explain.

Though it did sometimes happen that others were put before me for a booking on the basis of their association with others or particular professional establishments, I believed that this was surely, on most occasions, not the case. But I felt disheartened at my own personal situation preventing me from progressing as a creative professional for reasons that were entirely the result of unfortunate circumstance.

It was disheartening to know that I had very nearly come close several times, to being able to become part of the necessary professional organisations within the arts: I had at times been accepted by the establishments but had never been able to join them due to complete lack of the necessary funding or simply being in the wrong area.

This strange situation only continued; I was complimented by industry professionals and told that I made the grade in terms of, what they deemed to be talent. Yet these generous words were ultimately always followed with, 'But you just don't have enough of the professional training, nobody knows you and you are not a name.'

Much later I would suspect that a lack of being attached to something relevant or a name, has sometimes also held back some others who have been accepted within branches of the arts for their potential or talent but just were not known in any way. Perhaps, like me, they are not the kind of characters who get around these situations by pushing their way in or shouting about themselves, or by using others, but instead, simply want to focus on being able to do justice to any role or creative opportunity that we are fortunate enough to be given. Though I had ambition, I completely lacked in its entirety that ruthless type of it that I had seen in some, and which got them to where they felt that they were entitled to be. Rather, for me personally, I knew that I felt comfortable with the creative work that the professionals of the industry had told me I had something with and of which I felt such a connection to, and that was enough of a driving force: earning a living from something that feels natural to you and are kindly told that you have potential with, in a professional arena where you fit in is no bad thing. If only I could properly earn that living and in that way.

Although I went to every casting and meeting that I was told to when my painful symptoms allowed me to do so and did exactly as I was asked, always punctual and respectful of everyone, I found that, once again, the lack of opportunity in my earlier life and consequent lack of credentials and associates by way of being denied the professional training or not being in the right place to access being a part of one of the relevant professional establishments, was holding me back. But I would simply treat each situation, however disappointing in this respect, with good grace, always with politeness.

When I was sent for film or voiceover castings, nearly everyone in the castings and at the agencies came from London or the surrounding areas of the home counties and most had attended some kind of stage school or came to be in the profession by knowing someone, by way of living near to London. Many were pleasant, friendly people, and we got along fabulously. I would never tell them of my struggles, as I only ever wanted to be cheerful with people and, as I always knew, my situation was my own personal responsibility. But as I was told earlier in life, living in, or close to London meant having access to most of the opportunities required to become a professional within the arts. I was not from that part of the country and could not possibly afford to stay there at the time and therefore had never had any of the same opportunities.

An agent advised me that the more castings and auditions I did, the more that people within both the arts and modelling would get to know me and I would get bookings that way. But attending several castings or auditions a week would have cost hundreds of pounds each month in travel expenses – and I did not have that amount at the time - as they were nearly always in London. And I already knew that amount would be exceeded by far in the cost of living there. Even if your agency representation, whether for modelling or the arts, was outside of London, nearly all of the castings and bookings were there anyway.

I was constantly in a 'catch 22' situation: I needed to be continually attending castings and meetings in order for people in the industry to get to know me and to have a good chance of being able to become established professionally, but, the painful gynae symptoms that I had been experiencing for so long were preventing me from earning enough money to be able to fund travelling to, or staying in, London to do so.

Hardworking performers and creative artists who had not been to a performing arts school or were from other parts of the UK did break through occasionally, if they had access to sponsorship or living in another city that supported talent in the arts, such as Manchester. But the ratio swung almost entirely in favour of those living in or near to the capital, as in the home counties, at the time. That was not a fault of those living there, but rather that some places are just so overlooked when it comes to drawing talent for the creative industries. Where I had come from was particularly hopeless in this sense.

Though I was classed as being possibly an emerging talent, I was told that there was no way forward with this unless opportunity comes along. I spoke politely to the industry professionals when they struck-up conversation with me and the same thing would happen; they would often compliment me on some kind of talent that they saw in me (in this world of fabulously skilled performers however, I could not see that in myself, though I did at least feel competent at these professional fields and knew that I fitted-in well within them) or what a nice girl they thought me to be or so on. However, such compliments did not alter the fact that no matter how polite and punctual I was and how much I applied myself to what was expected of me, being unconnected and not living in, or near to, London, were, as I was told, the issues.

Though I had never let my unfortunate background be an excuse for anything or be any type of an issue, nevertheless, I found that having an optimistic attitude about that and being fully responsible for oneself is still not enough to overcome the practical issues faced with not being well-connected or living in an area where opportunities to progress in your profession are readily available.

But although many times I was disheartened to overhear others, who were not in need of the help that I was (and my circumstances had become apparent to some at times, however much I tried not to let them be an issue) be put in contact with people who could get them directly onto a booking, because of somebody that they were associated to, or given help to be in London and have access to bookings, auditions and castings. I never said anything about it because I absolutely do not want to hurt the feelings of others just because they have been more fortunate in life than me, especially as they had done nothing to me personally. They were not responsible for my circumstances, it was nobody's fault, and I understand that people can be oblivious to things at times, especially when they have no life experience of such matters themselves.

So, I just accepted the situation.

But foresight, instinct, and a good understanding of people is as imperative in this particular professional world as it is in others; it can lead to your noticing when someone is trying to do their best in life but is quietly struggling and needs a little help, and it can help us to see the possibilities of how far a person can take a good quality or skill and watch that grow. Sometimes it only takes one wise person with the means to do so to turn this situation on its head for the better. Humanity, I believe, can be enriched in mind, soul and character for it and it can lead to a knock-on effect where more good things come from that (something that I knew that if I ever did okay for myself in the future, I would implement to help others).

But as it was, I expected nothing from anyone.

I was perpetually stuck in this situation.

Feeling immensely downhearted, I began to wonder that this might not be meant to be. But I had been invited to become part of this arena from a young age for whatever they saw in my writing and performing and so the frequently positive feedback that I had received from the professionals within it, meant however, that logically, I was probably suitable for this professional world as a creative. I always thought that it was for others to decide if I have any talent at something, and, as I never had any actual bad feedback of any kind and with the enthusiastic recommendations that I had received, by that reasoning I thought I should perhaps not entirely give up on this route towards being a creative professional, simply through a lack of a pinch of good fortune. But whatever this bit of something good and interesting that some of these creative professionals had seen in me artistically, I did not know exactly what it was or what to do with it.

Instead, I felt like I was just muddling along, not really knowing what I was doing.

Thoughts of my writing arose again: I had written some concepts for film and tentatively showed these to a few others in the industry, but although they were enthusiastic about my writing style and the content of my work, they told me that because of my lack of a qualification in filmmaking or writing and with no TV experience or association to anything or anyone that was known, I would not be taken seriously if I proceeded to submit anything. 'It doesn't matter if you are a naturally skilled writer, like you are,' I was advised, 'you're completely unheard of, so nobody will be interested in publishing or producing your work.'

At times now, I felt desperate for relief from the pain and bleeding symptoms, but I kept my struggles to myself because I knew what would happen if I spoke to my doctor about them; I would be referred for embarrassing psychological assessments again. I had broken free of that, having been found to be of sound mind and with no troubling behavioural issues, but those particular professionals had wanted to continue to analyse me using the vague and unfounded reason of 'psychosomatic pain and bleeding caused by possible depression, possibly linked to childhood trauma'. Having been told, albeit subtly, that if I reported the 'psychosomatic' symptoms again, then they would have further power to intervene, I felt almost terrified by this.

Ethan advised me to raise the issue with the health service to see what could be done about my situation, but when I did so, I was merely informed that the cervical screening tests had shown definitively that I had no gynaecological illness and therefore the only clinical conclusion was that the symptoms were psychosomatic.

So, there was nothing more that I could do except cope with the pain.

It was then, however, that I began to be contacted more frequently for bookings and castings: some individuals had recognised my appeal, so I was told, and wanted to see what I could do. Finally, it seemed that I had just begun to break through the lack of stage school training, fame, and contacts issues, and was being seen simply for who I was as a creative and the work that I apparently had the ability to do.

Frustratingly, however, this did not turn out to be the good thing it should have been, as with the usual incredibly unfortunate timing in my life, the symptoms became worse and were severe at times—and such instances were becoming more and more frequent.

On the days where the symptoms seemed to be under control and manageable enough, I would head to London, portfolio in hand, travelling from tube station to tube station, as I attended the day's castings or auditions before catching the train for the journey back home. If my symptoms ever presented themselves on days like these—especially when I was travelling—it could prove quite disastrous for me if I found myself travelling in the middle of nowhere or on the tube, in pain and sometimes feeling like I was about to faint from the effects of the symptoms.

On one such occasion, with time to spare between castings, I exited the tube at Charing Cross Station and walked down to St James's Park, where I sat under a tree, trying to compose myself in the more peaceful surroundings in the hope that the pain would lessen. However, the pain did not ease, and so I sat in total frustration over my predicament, spending part of the afternoon simply trying to compose myself enough to be able to physically manage what was expected of me.

Regardless, I went along to my next casting looking pale, tired, and almost hobbling in pain, trying with every effort not to show the physical discomfort that I was in, which would not be taken kindly to at all, to say the least, in this particular professional environment, had I dared to reveal a little of what I was enduring. As usual back then, I seemed to encounter not particularly nice people who I would allow to order me around, because I did not dare rock the boat and answer back as they reminded me of their power, even without any reason for needing to do so.

Later though, on separate occasions, I would meet a few kind people in modelling. On one occasion, I was advised to attend an open call at one of London's most prominent agencies. Though I did not end up working with them as my look was not right for their particular requirements, where they were especially interested in very edgy looking runway models, the agent who I saw seemed to like something in my personality and self-expression. She sat with me, and studying my face, said 'you will get work with other agencies. You have some really pretty features.

Because of my long hair, I was often sent to castings for haircare commercials—usually in Kensington, Battersea or Chelsea. One of these such occasions was for a casting at the prestigious salon of a well-known hairdresser, and, at the sight of my tresses, he emerged from his office and ran his hands through it, gushing over how beautiful he thought it to be. I thought, from his enthusiastic reaction, that I might have that booking in the bag, but it was not to be, as the choosing of models had been delegated to a casting team who decided that only models from London should be booked.

But more hair castings for other companies slowly came my way, and I was also booked for a shoot at a major haircare company at their headquarters. This was a well-paid booking—but, once again, I was overcome by the mystery pelvic pain. Hence, it materialised that I could not make the booking because of this.

Some of the other booking or casting requests that I could not attend as a result of my health issue had interesting elements to them—fun and stylish things. On one occasion, I was taken aback by my receiving a lovely email complimenting my look, accompanied with a booking request, from the charming head of Fashion TV, who had selected me to walk in a show for a label. The booking was not for a famous designer (I was absolutely never anywhere near established as a model for that and also, though I did have a good walk, it was commercial modelling that my look was more suited to) but the kind and unexpected email was nice to receive, and I responded that I would be happy to accept the request.

'There will be at least some labels who will see you if you do the show, and, with your great walk, there is a possibility that you might be given more work,' I was told by a casting agent.

I certainly did not think that I could be a top model by any means but that did not matter as it was never about that for me; modelling was only one small aspect of what I could do and I only intended for it to be a means to an end to hopefully provide the funding that I needed to establish my work as a creative within the arts. So I gratefully accepted opportunities because, having been invited into this arena, not only did I enjoy some of the creative aspects of photography and fashion, but I also thought they might at least help me to get out of my increasingly difficult circumstances if I could go on to earn a decent living.

Hence, I arranged to travel to London for fittings—only for it to happen *again*: the symptoms became severe and attempting to manage them with over-the-counter pain relief, early on the day of the booking, I tried to get myself ready for my commute to London, despite the fact that I was almost doubled over in pain. I knew that I would not even be able to make it to the train station in such a state and consequently had to call those I was due to work with and let them know that I could not make it.

I lost the booking—one of many that I had already lost, because of the symptoms.

I would never have the chance to explain to the Fashion TV people, nor those from the labels who had shown a little interest in working with me, that as it would turn out many years later, that I had been suffering from cancer at the time. The opportunities that had been presented to me in the world of fashion had just been lost forever.

6
Falling Apart

AS THE PAINFUL PELVIC SYMPTOMS steadily escalated, my quality of life, declined progressively over the years, as the pain frequently interrupted my ability to work consistently, and as a by-product I now had no social life at all and no material comforts. Ethan had problems of his own, too: he was finding it incredibly difficult to manage the problems he was facing since his service in the military, and he desperately needed help, particularly with obtaining his civilian further education to enter a new profession but was turned away from all assistance and received none whatsoever. Hence, he bravely continued with the circumstances of his life as best he could—and did a sterling job of it, too, always working so hard and being completely independent. I looked after him as much as I could—we both tried to help each other—but we were both faced with overwhelming obstacles that could not be improved simply by putting all our own efforts into fixing them and being optimistic.

Out of desperation, and with fear that I might be again sent for even further psychoanalyses or that more intense action might be taken by trying to force me into some kind of therapy or anti-depressants, I made a last-ditch attempt to politely plead with a new doctor to help me with the pelvic pain. But she would only listen to the other doctors' opinion, written in my medical notes, that these symptoms had been deemed psychosomatic and therefore said that she would have to report my complaining of the symptoms again to the psychological health department. Now too frightened to further speak of them again because of this, that was the last time I ever told a doctor of the pain symptoms.

What am I going to do? Why won't the doctors believe me? Is this ever going to end? I would ruminate in despair. I knew now for sure that it would be entirely futile to seek medical help again for my gynae symptoms—and, even worse than that, I knew that if I did so once more, having been told in no uncertain terms that seeking medical help for my symptoms would no longer be possible and would almost certainly lead to me being forced into further psychological analyses and possibly forced intervention of anti-depressants on the basis of, as they had been deemed at the time, psycho-somatic symptoms that may possibly be due to depression. I was too afraid to ever mention what I was going through to any doctor ever again.

It was during this time—when my life was slowly but surely worsening due to the gynae symptoms—that I began gaining some actual professional interest as a creative and a little for modelling.

Those in the industry weren't entirely put off by my having to turn down bookings and castings due to my physical symptoms just yet, as further interesting requests began to arrive. My lack of being known or well-connected seemed to become slowly less important to those in the industry as people were beginning to get to know me a little and apparently liked what they saw in doing so, and more and more booking and casting requests slowly came my way.

Would I accept a booking for a walk-on, small speaking role in a popular British TV programme? I did not watch the show—it was not really my thing—but I had heard it mentioned many times due to its popularity. It was far from my ideal choice of booking or career—being on TV never interested me and it was not what I want to do—but I was in dire circumstances financially and needed to earn a living and therefore grateful of the opportunity.

Though I had not put myself forward for the role, the casting people of the show had selected me for a very minor part, especially after seeing some of my portfolio and hearing my voice.

'Thank you for booking me, but you should know that I am not an actress,' I responded cordially. However, they were not put off by this as they wanted to see how my presence on-screen might translate.

Although my symptoms were now very troublesome, I had been able to complete what was asked of me professionally when I could get the symptoms under control for a little while, so maybe this would be a time when I could get a booking done without the symptoms disrupting things too much.

But sure enough, the pelvic pain grew in severity yet again, and the evening that I was due to travel to the location for early-morning filming, I could hardly walk as a result of the degree of my discomfort. Over-the-counter pain relief was doing little to take the sharp pains away this time.

I deliberated over continuing with the booking, since I foresaw the likelihood of my turning up at the location in a pained state and ultimately disrupting the filming schedule due to my being incapacitated by my symptoms.

So, just like the other times before now, I reluctantly and disappointedly had to call in and turn the booking down.

Another time, an exciting booking request arrived involving the music world: 'You would look fantastic in this video that I am shooting for a band. We need a great model for this, but someone who can dance really well and you're a professional dancer so perfect! Could you make it to location next week?'

Could I ever! But what was I going to do about the pain symptoms? Enthused at the prospect of being involved with the artistic aspects of music and film, I was not interested in the actual being seen on camera, though knew that was essentially what I was being booked for, it was more that I simply loved the creativity surrounding it. So I agreed to the booking, thinking that I could control the symptoms with over-the-counter pain relief to enable me to do the work. But as the day came around, I found myself sitting on the bathroom floor, with my arms wrapped around my abdomen, fruitlessly attempting to get the pain under control.

Other castings and bookings that I had to turn down, always for the very same reason, were further dance bookings for film, sitting for artists as a muse and voice work.

After all of that time of struggling to get anywhere with my creative work due to not having any start in the arts, as I had been recommended for, simply due to lack of funding, things had subtly begun to turn the other way as I had been tenacious with that particular struggle—and yet all of the booking requests that I was now receiving were scuppered by my symptoms.

But while I did manage to be able to cope with the pain enough in order to accept a few of these requests, I ended up missing many as a result of the painful symptoms—most of which being interesting, well-paid bookings.

Seeing my professional prospects disappearing into thin air because of issues that I could not seem to do anything about, no matter how hard I tried, was a frustrating situation.

How could I stop this downward spiral? Would I ever be free from this mysterious condition that was causing me—and, consequently, Ethan—considerable suffering?   I   was perpetually trapped by circumstance. I had always thought that it was all down to me to make the most of my life, but no matter how much I tried to live my life correctly, work hard, do all of the right things, and treat others respectfully, nothing that I did would ever alter the course of my life in any progressive or healthy way.

Being unable to attend many bookings now, meant that I had to try other types of work that I could manage around the effects of the pelvic symptoms in order to try and survive financially and I began to veer off the professional path that I had been almost placed on early in life. Some people who I vaguely knew through the business saw other skills in me in the form of (apparently) qualities that they could utilise. This included a little of assisting briefly in the creative side of modelling and the arts for would-be artists and models who had a great deal of financial backing and support but needed skilled people around them to mould their careers. But I found myself repeatedly messed around by them and once again, it was difficult to actually get them to pay me for anything that I did.

On one such occasion, I was asked to help a woman from a prestigious background, regarding her forthcoming music promotion. After being told how trustworthy and sensible I was and how I had been deemed to have some potential talent as a creative, she was keen to have me on her team to shape the image aspect of the musical career that she wanted to obtain, though I was mystified as to why as I was not part of the music industry and never had been. She seemed to want to compete with her celebrity friend and was hellbent on becoming a famous singer and attaining a chart hit (though, as it would turn out, this would never come to fruition).

The woman told me that with my lack of connections, I was unlikely to ever become anything as a creative—though she suggested that I should try to become a TV presenter, like someone else that she personally knew, because she felt that I had a distinctive voice style, along with an articulate way of speaking. However, she added that I was not to think I could ever really do anything with that due to my not being from the 'right type of background or connected'. Before I could respond to say that I did not want to be a TV Presenter, she suddenly announced, however, that she would refuse to help me, as she thought that people should not use connections and should instead make it on their own.

Though baffled by this ironic statement from someone who did not appreciate that she had been fortunate enough never to have to do anything alone or without help her whole life, I simply responded diplomatically, 'thank you for the compliments on my voice and the advice, but I am not interested in being on TV. Voice, yes; in person, no'. before politely adding, 'and you need not concern yourself that I might ask you for anything. I have barely ever asked anyone for help for anything in my life. I have met prominent people since my teens and never asked any of them for anything.'

The fact that *she* had come to *me* for help had completely escaped her.

I began to feel dispirited that having, apparently, the suitability for the arts and entertainment industries as a professional myself, was nevertheless unable to progress in this field as a result of the persistence of my physical symptoms and particular deprived circumstances—making my being treated the way that I was for not having the same good fortune in life as some others all the more disheartening. I was happy for them but found their rudeness and ignorance difficult to tolerate.

In the midst of my decline, my health began to take a new, somewhat strange turn, and the doctors agreed, though unwillingly, with the wishes of the nice hospital doctor who had suspected that I was genuinely suffering from a physical issue, to at this point keep an eye on the functioning of my body through bloodwork due to my slightly increased white blood cell levels.

This time, the blood test showed the usual slightly raised white blood cells but now possessed a new feature: elevated levels of a particular hormone. The doctor explained to me that such results were indicative of a certain type of brain tumour and told me that he would arrange a referral to a neurologist at the local hospital.

To the doctors' surprises however, the results of my head scan came back normal: no brain tumour.

The elevated hormone level was not investigated any further. Later, however, it would transpire to be a possible indicator of what was going on with my health.

The persistent and worsening symptoms of pain and bleeding, however, were still impacting me severely. I was relieved to still be able to exercise and work on the occasions when the pain was not so bad—partially through medicating it heavily with over-the-counter analgesics, although these remedies never caused the pain to fully dissipate. The problem was not going to go away, and I could never speak of this again to a doctor because of what had been wrongly stated in my medical notes about the symptoms being psycho-somatic: if I did so, I would henceforth (wrongly) be viewed as needing more psychological analyses and forced anti-depressant treatment. Hence, all I could do was live with the misery my symptoms instilled in me and keep trying my best; keep plodding on; keep working hard through the pain; keep watching my life break down into nothing, until I might well find myself homeless. I berated myself constantly for not being able to get myself out of the situation that I was in.

Booking or casting enquiries did still happen on occasion; it had not all entirely slipped through my fingers, due to my circumstances, just yet.

A professional on a casting for a commercial approached me, took my details, and emailed me out of the blue with an opportunity to meet with a London acting agency to see if they would be interested in representing me based on the skills that I was apparently seen to have, despite my lack of being established as an artist. I had explained that I did not think of myself as an actress and wasn't particularly interested in being one (that being because I thought it was a profession that I could never be good enough for), and though people had suggested to me that I should try acting, I felt that I might be better suited to using my voice. But she insisted that I possibly had something appealing for acting work and so encouraged me to meet with the agency with whom I could also try out for voicework.

Though, despite being told from a young age by some in the industry that I had something of a natural basis for acting, I could not envision myself at all as an actress—especially as all of the actors whose work I enjoyed were spectacularly talented—nor had any intention to become one, I thought it would be terribly ungrateful of me to turn down such an opportunity, as well as it being a chance to perhaps go on to earn a bit of money. As I had previously been working on bits and pieces of writing for script, I reasoned that if I made the grade, my experience with the acting agency might enable me to find my place either as a performer or a writer—or, if I was really lucky, as both. Perhaps eventually this would enable me to earn some of the credentials needed that I had been lacking due to circumstance.

But I had no idea how I was going to manage the pelvic pain enough to be consistent with the work.

Over the course of the next couple of months, I was asked to record a few pieces, as well as to attend some castings. The pelvic symptoms were sometimes bearable enough for me to do so. One of the casting professionals that I encountered here seemed quite delighted with me. 'They loved you, Rebecka! We've had great feedback about you, but they need further discussion, and we won't know their decision for some weeks.'

It looked like there might be a tiny possibility that I had done something okay as a potential performer and that this might lead to more work professionally and for me that would mean a boosted income and perhaps lead to the opportunity to progress as a creative.

A couple of weeks later, I was told that I had not got the part that I was sent for. Of course, I could absolutely take this in my stride—many of the bookings that any model, dancer, actor or performer cast for they don't get, and rejection is part of the business. However, learning that I had been unsuccessful in the casting not due to any lack of the required skill or because of any unsuitability was something I felt I could learn from. I didn't mind criticism and have found that in most areas of my life, it can often be good to especially listen to the constructive type of it. 'Did they say anything in terms of how I could improve? If I have done badly at something, I would like to know, so that I can correct it,' I had asked my booker.

She responded, 'you did nothing wrong. You actually did everything really well. But you are just not known at all so it would be a risk for them to take a chance on you.'

I completely accepted this information and took it on board. But I wondered how on Earth I could solve the glaring problem of not being able to become an established artist if I already had to *be* one to work on anything. I felt that perhaps I would be better off just sticking to my writing, but with that, of course, I faced a similar problem: being completely unknown.

But that had never factored into it when I got into this profession. It was only the art of it that interested me.

Despite these wonderings, I did manage to make it to a few more castings, as well as the occasional booking, around my ever-worsening symptoms. Nobody in the castings ever had any clue that I was in so much discomfort: eternally well-prepared, I was always on time and had already read through anything the booker, client, or agent wanted me to beforehand, was always polite to everyone, and would do exactly what was asked of me, the whole time trying to sufficiently manage the pain.

Sometimes, I was devastated upon receiving a booking with a good fee for a day's work and having to turn such prospects down, being in too much pain to go through with it. Indeed, for a number of years now, the situation with my symptoms had steadily robbed Ethan and I of the possible financial stability we had tried so hard and from such a young age to achieve. A never-ending cycle of deprivation continued for both of us, and it never eased—only worsened.

It was around this time that I had a very strange experience with my fledgling creative work whereby some businesspeople, with a connection to show businesses and the media, had taken quite an interest in me after seeing some of my images and hearing about how apparently I had some kind of appeal, which I later discovered they were trying to exploit to promote their business interests. Fortunately, this matter did not go far: it was swiftly dealt with by the appropriate authorities. This saga did, however, add to my continual problem of others trying to take advantage of (what I did not know at the time to be) my perilous circumstances.

This incident was one of many where over the coming years, I began to attract even more unscrupulous people than usual. When a person is falling to their lowest point, they can sometimes let their guard down and become mistreated in a number of ways.

The verbal abuse, mainly by women, that I had faced in my area also continued almost whenever I left the house and succeeded in making me nervous.

Men were often nice to me, but sometimes I was followed and harassed by others. 'I could have you if I wanted to', I was told on a few occasions, while a couple of times I was left shaken-up when they tried to almost pull me into their cars.

Ethan and others had told me that I was unusual in a place such as where we lived and so some people there sometimes reacted to this in over-the-top ways.

I desperately wanted to leave the place because I wanted to get away from the daily abuse that I received for not fitting in there, but to be able to move home, I would need to earn much more money—a task that was becoming more and more impossible because of how the painful pelvic symptoms were disrupting my life.

There are some nice parts of the area and also certainly some absolutely lovely and genial people there and it would be good if that was the focal point, as they are the redeeming factors.

However, entirely separately from that, in regard to many others of a particular attitude, there was hatred and shaming towards attributes in a person. Being understanding and polite and friendly didn't make any difference and you couldn't reason with them in any way.

There is no gentler way of describing it, but there were also some who had been overindulged and shown no boundaries and for whom little expectation was placed on personal responsibility (something I would unwittingly notice throughout my life time and can appear in all areas of society, and I expect that others have noticed as such too), leading to them acquiring an astonishing sense of entitlement and no real regard for the wellbeing of others. This was apparent as they made a misery of the lives of those who had to live around them; mindless behaviour that is enabled by excuses being made for its presence (along with, like other places, rife narcotic drug use in particular areas).

Why is there, I wonder, an obligation for us to love where we come from, even if that place is unhealthy for us and we could never fit in there, where we could never truly belong or be ourselves?

Being able to publish my writing would have gone some way to helping get me out of the circumstances that I was stuck in and trying with every effort to get myself out of, but although my written pieces were accepted as being of the necessary standards, nevertheless, I was always told that as an unknown, I would never be able to get any further with this.

Will I ever get out of this situation? I wondered. I was never going to receive treatment for my symptoms, and so therefore would very likely always suffer from them. I kept telling myself that I needed to find a way through this; of managing my symptoms so that I could salvage my work. After all, earning a living seemed to be the only way out of this. However, deep down, I knew that life was to simply continue in this existence. My symptoms were worsening, and I began to find myself in penurious circumstances due to the symptoms frequently interrupting my being able to work and my consequently lacking the earnings that I should have been getting for the jobs that I was booked for but could not do most of because of the pelvic pain. We were starting to fear that we may be forced to sell the house—but this would effectively leave us homeless and as we had nowhere to go to and the monthly payments on the mortgage cost the same amount as rent would in any case, selling the house would make no difference.

Hence, as we at least had somewhere to live, we started to go without basic material needs to prioritise keeping our home.

Life got harder, and the painful symptoms continued to increase steadily. It was around this time that at a casting I was referred to an agency run by a gracious woman who was nice to me.

I managed to do a couple more castings, including for the performing arts agency. Though I was never intending to be an actress, having been unexpectedly so ushered into that world I felt that in this arena I could at least make use of my voice and my understanding of movement and physicality, so I thought I should accept the opportunity. I had previously scraped together what little money I had left to fund the travel expenses required for castings but by now, I no longer had any means whatsoever to fund travel to them and so that issue along with the extremely troublesome pelvic symptoms, meant that I had to stop attending castings.

If I could just permanently deal with my physical health problem, I thought, I might be on the way to getting somewhere with my creative work or perhaps as a model. But though I tried to cope with it, the pain was becoming more unbearable.

Mostly, I was finding it difficult to function at all: the pelvic pain was by now almost constant, and despite my desperate attempts to continue as normal, ultimately, I found that I could not attend any of the bookings that I was being offered.

Little did I know that just as I joined the agencies who were offering me the work that had the potential to provide the professional breakthrough that I had needed, at exactly the same time, my life was about to take a dramatic turn in events on a scale that I could never have possibly imagined.

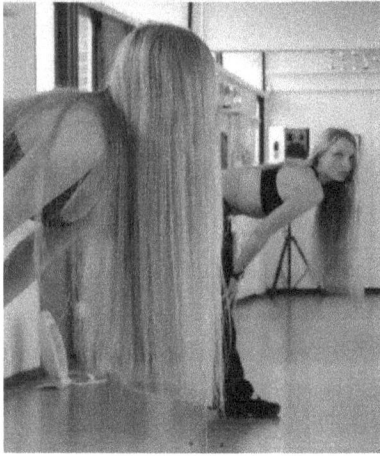

A mirror image, training in the dance studio

Photo Credit: R.B

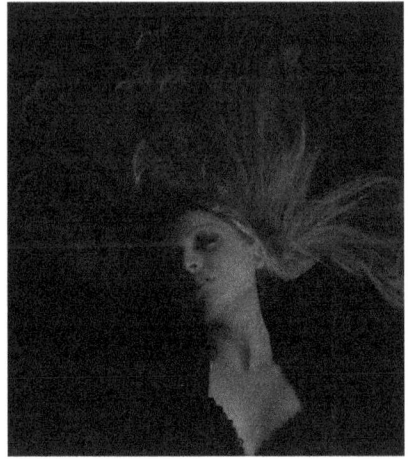

An artistic modelling shot, meant to capture the apparently 'ethereal' look and hair that I was deemed to have.

Photo Credit: R.B

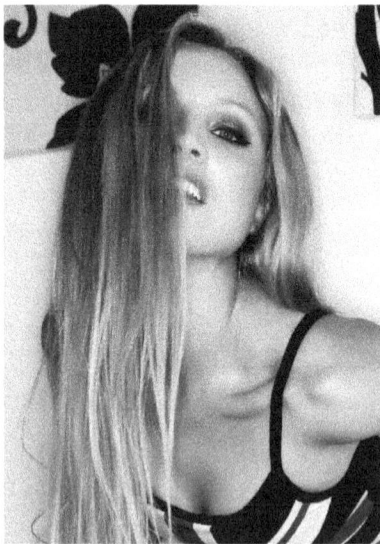

Photo Credit: LeSauvage

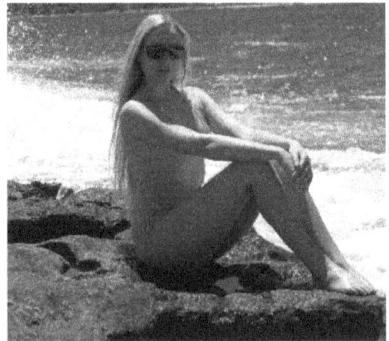

Photo Credit: B.B

7
An Unusual Case

WHAT HAD HAPPENED TO ME so far did not form the darkest part of my life. The darker, most sickening parts were about to come—and they began like this, one August day, with a letter that arrived in the post.

It was a routine letter, sent to nearly all women in England every three years or so: *Your cervical screening test is due. Please call your local health surgery to book your appointment.* The letter, of course, had no effect on me: I was not surprised or concerned by it, since it was simply a routine test and standard letter and identical to those that I had received many times before in the preceding years, and which, continuously being so responsible for my health, I always took serious notice of. Hence, as always, I booked the test appointment as soon as I was requested to, always being sure never to miss any.

When the day of the test arrived, carried out with the nurse at my local medical practice, it materialised that the nurse could not perform the test, as she found that there seemed to be an issue preventing her from doing so; something was not quite right with my body.

'It's probably nothing to worry about,' said the nurse, 'but I'm going to refer you to the female doctor; she knows more about these situations than me.'

I did not worry about any serious medical issue; chronic, probably, but life-threatening, no.

A few days later, I walked from my home to the medical practice to attend for the test appointment—the one with the female doctor.

As I walked up the road, three women, perhaps in their late twenties, were standing at a bus stop and caught sight of me walking in their direction. They began shouting at me in their regional-English accent. There are some British regional accents that are very likeable and which I find charming, but, simply in the observational sense and not a mocking one, there are others that can perhaps, in their heaviest form, be not to everyone's taste or challenging to follow. Interestingly, these kinds of women of a particular type of personality and character who were now shouting at me were the very ones who, where I came from, repeatedly aggressively mocked my elocution.

'Oh. Oh, look at 'er!' one of them shouted to her companions.

Their loud discussion revealed that they were encouraging each other to physically intimidate me.

Normally, I would have turned and gone on an alternate route at the realisation that I was entering a volatile situation, but on this occasion, the meaning of my journey was far too important to do so. Therefore, I nervously walked past the cackling aggressive trio.

'Look at 'ow she walks! Oh, look at what she's wearin'! 'Oo does she think she is?' another jeered.

'Oh, *look* at the silly bitch,' one of the instigators mockingly shouted as I walked past, then became more aggrieved, 'Oi, don't ignore me, yer' silly bitch. I'll punch yer if yer walk through ere' again', they shouted at the top of their voice.

The apparent offensive way in which I walked was simply due to good posture, mostly due to dance training, while the offending clothes were perceived so simply because they were perhaps feminine.

The jeering perpetrators did not seem to realise that if they had spoken to me normally, I would have responded and in a friendly manner.

Regardless, the screeching and jeering continued as I walked past feeling embarrassed and harassed, trying to focus only on the view ahead. But thankfully the screeching women did not make physical contact with me, and I arrived at the medical practice unscathed.

The doctor tried to begin the test upon my arrival—only to find it very difficult to do so. She was most concerned and diligent as she examined me more thoroughly, saying that she was not happy with just a simple examination as she wanted to be absolutely sure that there was no serious health issue.' She suddenly went quiet. She pulled up a chair beside me. 'Rebecka,' she said in a very calm voice, 'I have found something. You have a tumour on your cervix.'

I tried to absorb this sudden, new, and daunting information 'Okay.' I paused calmly. 'What happens now?'

The doctor did not panic me at all and sat for a couple of minutes beside me, a soft, reassuring smile on her face and her voice gentle. 'Well, I managed to get a tiny sample of the surrounding tissue cells,' she explained. 'I am sending that off to the lab today, and then I'm going to make an urgent referral for you to the gynae-oncology department.' She was very reassuring but firm. 'We need to get this sorted right away.'

With this diagnosis, I left the medical practice and walked home in pain. To make matters worse, I could see from a distance that the same women were still at the bus stop. I crossed to the opposite side of the street in order to avoid them, but they continued their tirade, and this verbal abuse, that I had become used to, now felt even worse to receive in this particularly distressing and painful moment. They attempted to cross the road to follow me, but I got out of their way as quickly as I could.

Upon reaching home, I lay on the sofa in pain and calmly pondered over the doctor's findings. Ethan was at work. When he returned home that evening, I told him about my news. Neither of us were particularly upset or frightened; we are generally very pragmatic people. 'You've been here before, remember?' Ethan pointed out. 'With a breast tumour, which was benign. Then they thought you had a brain tumour, and it turned out you didn't. There's something physically wrong obviously, but it's most probably nothing serious.'

Yes, that makes sense, I thought. *As before, it's probably nothing to worry about.*

However, the next day, another Doctor called me; the tissue sample that had been taken in the test the day before had been flagged up by the lab with urgency and showing that I had an established, high-grade cancer of the cervix. I was to be sent to the gynaecology-oncology department of my local hospital the following morning.

But how can I have cervical cancer when I have never missed a cervical screening test? I thought, *and not only that but all the tests had been shown as normal.* It was then that I had a sudden thought: the symptoms that I had suffered with for many years seemed to fit with those of cervical cancer. However, I rationalised that surely the tests for cervical cancer would have picked that up years previously.

Four days after attending the test, I found myself sitting in the waiting room of a hospital gynae-oncology department.

As we waited to be called for my appointment, I wondered what would happen, concluding that perhaps it was better to wait until I had been examined by the gynae-oncologist and receive his diagnosis before worrying much about the situation.

A nurse specialist called me into a room where a consultant introduced himself and seemed surprised at the sight of me. He stared inquisitively as I shook his hand.

He informed me that—in complete contrast to what the doctors had previously told me, in being referred as a matter of urgency—I had been referred to him as a precaution. As we engaged in conversation, I noticed that he seemed to be studying my appearance a fair bit, but I was used to people doing that, so did not read too much into it. He seemed pleasant and friendly enough but said something a little odd, given the content of the phone call that I had received from the doctor two days earlier.

'I can absolutely tell you that you don't have cancer.'

I paused. 'But I don't understand. The tests results...'

'They don't necessarily mean anything,' he replied simply. Ethan looked instantly relieved, but although I did not express it, I could not see the logic behind why the doctor would have told me over the phone that not only had my test result been positive, but that it had also shown that I had a high-grade form of cervical cancer.

This is odd, I thought, but I did not stress about it, *this gentleman is an expert of his professional field. If anyone is going to know the exactitude of the test result, surely it's going to be him.*

With that, the consultant went on to tell me that he would give me an examination anyway just to check that there were no issues. The examination was painful. Once this was completed, the consultant said, 'There may be a slight issue with inflammation, but nothing serious. Just normal gynaecological issues; definitely not cancer. However, just as a matter of routine, the nurse specialist will arrange for you to be booked into the surgical ward over the next few days so that I can examine you under anaesthetic.'

As I stood up to leave, he added, 'I can *absolutely* assure you that you do *not* have cancer.'

But the hugely differing opinions of the doctors regrading my most recent test results did not make sense. After all, why would the female doctor tell me that she had found a tumour, and then the doctor who called me tell me that my test results had shown that I had cancer, if neither of these were true? Could I trust the consultant's opinion? *Of course I can,* I reasoned, *as he is the specialist, after all.*

Three days later, I was in a hospital ward, preparing to have explorative gynaecological surgery under anaesthetic.

When the nurses had left the ward for a few minutes, I noticed they had left a folder of my medical records sitting on the bed. I stared at the folder, realising that I had never read my medical records before—and I had a deep feeling that I could learn what was going on by seeing for myself the information regarding my cancer diagnosis. So, inquisitively, I reached for and opened the bundle of documents.

I was surprised to read comments referring to an apparent history of possible depression, the onset of which only being mentioned when I reported the symptoms of what now seemed to be due to a tumour, (partly written by my new gynae-oncology consultant, who had only just met me), referring to what was deemed a manifestation of itself in the form of repeated reporting of psychosomatic pain and bleeding. Alongside these reports were comments from when I had been forced to see the psychological health professionals on the basis of there being no other explanation for my gynaecological symptoms, dating back to when I first began to report them, stating 'possible depression' as the cause of 'psychosomatic' gynaecological symptoms. But this one statement had been enough to completely change the course of how I was viewed and I was completely unaware that my medical care could be so influenced by one opinion, especially one from someone who is not an expert of female health or oncological care; the opinion being, essentially, that having discovered, through asking about my childhood, that I was from a harsh and abusive early life and with the cervical screening results all being stated as normal, the gynae symptoms must therefore be psychological because of my deprived early start—this opinion was upheld even though I was in hospital right at that moment, being treated for the pain and bleeding after receiving test results confirming cervical cancer.

While scanning the records for some information regarding my previous screening test results, I was beginning to read about this when I glanced up to find the consultant who I had seen a couple of days earlier looking at me with a serious expression, holding out his hand for me to give him the notes.

He hastily took them from me. I remained polite but couldn't help feeling that there was something not quite right in all of this, especially as the dates of the tests had been over the same time period as my reporting of the pain and bleeding symptoms.

Later, back on the ward after the surgery, the nurses roused me from my anaesthetic-induced slumber. 'Sleeping Beauty,' one said to the other, just as I opened my eyes, to find them sweetly gazing at me. They talked me through how the surgery had gone, explaining that the surgeon had removed a small part of my cervix for testing and that the findings would not be known for a few days, but that that he did not think there was anything at all to worry about other than perhaps some common gynaecological problems, if even that. I was also informed that the nature of the surgery meant that there would be significant bleeding, and so the theatre team had secured a gauze 'pack' internally, which would stay in place for several hours. Otherwise, there had apparently been no issues, and I could be discharged in a few hours.

When they later came to remove the 'pack', a most undignified procedure indeed, I cried out in agony as reams of fabric were ripped (they have to do this fast and with force, apparently, so that nothing gets accidentally left behind) from my fresh internal wound. Physical pain was something that I had no choice but to adapt to throughout my life and I was accustomed to it, so for me to even flinch at something means it is causing severe pain—and yet here, I cried out aloud.

I lay writhing in pain on the hospital bed—and, upon finding me in such acute discomfort, the nurses decided to keep me in overnight.

The next morning, I tried to get out of bed. 'Come on, come and get ready to go home,' said a nurse. I could barely move for the pain. 'Oh, you young girls, feeling sorry for yourselves' she sighed. Though the date of birth of a patient is written on their hospital wristband and notes, this is not always seen unless the nurses specifically have to look at that information, and, given that I always looked so much younger than my age, the nurse, like most other people, treated me as a teenager. 'Come on, get up, we need to discharge you.'

Lying on my side, I edged off the bed but could hardly lift my legs off of it and winced as I tried to place my feet on the floor. The nurse's previously jovial facial expression but mildly irritated manner suddenly became serious. 'Goodness, you really *are* in a lot of pain, aren't you?' she said as she took me by the arm and got me to my feet. With that, I walked to the bathroom, which was incredibly painful to do.

The nurse's station was by the bathroom and as their shift was changing from the night to the morning, they were giving the morning staff a brief of updates and details on the patients in their care. As I hobbled towards the bathroom door, they had not noticed me or the trail of blood pooling on the floor from where I had walked as they had their briefing.

I had got a shock when I went to use the bathroom.

Then, as I headed back out to get help from the nurses, I overheard the nurse giving the meeting say, 'Rebecka has been assessed by a psychiatrist and has been found to have psychosomatic gynaecological pain and bleeding due to possible depression.'

I was perplexed to hear these words regarding that assessment many years before. I wanted to explain to them that the only reason I had received those assessments at all was that it had been assumed that the pain and bleeding were psychosomatic when no other clinical explanation could be found. It briefly occurred to me, amidst the extreme pain that I was in, that this may have been why some of the nurses had been sharp with me or had frequently brushed off my pain.

But right now, I had something far more urgent that needed attending to.

'I am sorry to interrupt,' I quietly intercepted the nurses' meeting, 'but I have a problem.'

'What's wrong?' asked one of the nurses.

'I'm bleeding fairly severely.'

'*No*, you're not Rebecka,' replied the nurse, exasperated.

'Please, I really am,' I begged. 'I am bleeding. I am bleeding *badly*.' I revealed my blood-soaked nightdress and the blood all over the floor, and with that, the nurses sprang into action, taking me into the bathroom, where they were surprised to find such a large amount of blood.

The nurses gave me some dressings and, I painfully hobbled back to the hospital bed. But a new nurse came onto shift and abruptly told me, 'Right, you have to be discharged now.'

'Please, I don't like to complain about pain, but I'm really in agony...' I wincingly tried to explain.

But my pleas fell upon deaf ears, as I received nothing but a scolding for what the nurse saw as time-wasting. It seemed she had believed in the validity of the assigned 'psychosomatic' label to explain my reporting of the symptoms, and, sure enough, went on to state this to her colleague.

Just ten minutes later, another nurse came to me and said that my gynaecologist-oncologist consultant had asked to speak to me in a side office, which I was then led to tentatively, in great pain. The nurse who had just scolded me was sat in the office and smiled warmly at me as I tentatively stepped into the room, wearing a hospital gown. Such a sudden complete change in attitude seemed really peculiar. The consultant told me to take a seat. The nurse's behaviour towards me had drastically changed to kindness.

The consultant addressed me, 'We have had the results back of the tissue samples that we took in the surgery, and we have found something: you have a tumour.'

'A benign tumour?' I asked. Having had benign tumours in the past, I assumed this would just be another. But it also occurred to me that the doctor who had called me had already diagnosed me with a high-grade cancer, despite the new Gynae-oncologist stating otherwise, so I wanted to be absolutely sure of the tumour's status.

'No. A cancerous tumour,' the consultant answered.

'I have cancer?'

'Yes,' the doctor replied.

I felt suddenly overwhelmed of the knock-on effects of the illness on my life, such as how Ethan would manage, the prospect of having the mortgage to pay with only one salary and the effect of the illness and treatment on the possibility of my being able to progress as a creative and therefore finally improve my life. I welled up at the thought of all of this, and the consultant held my hand.

It seemed like an act of compassion, which I appreciated. But I was puzzled at why he had previously been so insistent on saying that my pain and bleeding was all in my mind when it had been glaringly obvious by this stage that it was not. How could he have been so convinced, with all the evidence and opinions of the doctors that were new to my case and were stating a diagnosis of cancer, that I was not suffering from that and must surely instead have depression, as the psychiatrist had stated? It did not make sense.

What did make sense now, however, was that I was in such pain and had lost such a large amount of blood after the surgery and had been in such agony with the 'pack' being removed, because there was an actual growing tumour present and a high-grade cancerous one at that.

We chatted for a while about how the cancer would be treated, and they informed me that a multidisciplinary team meeting was required for my complex case of cancer so that all those involved in my care could discuss the best way forward.

The consultant stood, shook my hand, and said goodbye as he headed for the door. But, before he could leave, something profoundly logical suddenly occurred to me: *How on Earth can I have cervical cancer when I have never missed a screening test, and all the other tests had shown to be normal?* I suddenly voiced this question, to which the consultant answered crassly a surprising response: 'Well, Rebecka, you know... *shit happens.*'

As the late summer weather bathed England in glistening sunshine, I recovered from the surgery. The surgical bleeding, by way of cutting into the tumour and removing some of the cervix, had continued, but just as the consultant had expected, it gradually lessened. The surgical pain also lessened as the wound healed, but, of course, the pain from the tumour remained as a result of what we now knew it to be—cancer—and so until that was gone, the pain would never go away.

There was no fuss or drama surrounding my cancer diagnosis. I hardly told anyone about it and simply got on with my life as though nothing had happened: I had to.

Over the next few weeks, there were a variety of meetings held by the MDT, and I received letters, and phone calls every now and then to inform me of the outcome of them.

I was sent for a scan to facilitate the doctors' determining of the exact position of my tumour. As we sat in the semi-full waiting room of the scan department, with some of the patients looking anxious as they awaited their tests, a TV blared away in the corner with a dreary British soap opera. Few were paying attention to it, and some were as irritated by it as I was. I found myself drily observing to Ethan, 'Gosh, that programme is more depressing than my cancer.' Most of the patients and their families, and also Ethan, burst out into laughter as I smiled warmly at them. There is a time and a place for both seriousness and humour, and where appropriate, to elicit a moment's lightness for people from life's harsher realities.

Weeks passed, and during that time, my test results came back, determining how the cancer was growing and how it was affecting the way that my body was functioning, and which the doctors discussed amongst themselves. My nurse specialist and gynaecologist-oncologist consultant explained to me that the test results had shown some unusual growth in the tumour in terms of its position and direction of spread. The unusual properties of my particular case made me unsuitable for treatment at my local hospital and I would instead require very specialised care. For that reason, I would be referred to a highly skilled surgeon who specialised in this field at a medical establishment situated in another part of England. The area in which it was situated was completely unfamiliar to Ethan and me. The Royal Marsden cancer hospital, however, is a renowned hospital based in central London and we both knew London very well, so I asked if it would be possible to receive my treatment there.

An enquiry was made on my behalf with the appropriate surgeon at the Royal Marsden Hospital, and all three teams from the three different medical establishments would then hold meetings and correspond with one another regarding the best way forward with my treatment. My case of cancer was rather complicated, I was informed, and treating it would require liaising, opinion and planning between the different teams.

Autumn arrived, and a month and a half passed since my initial surgery. An appointment arrived for me to see an eminent surgeon at the medical establishment that my consultant had mentioned. Ethan and I attended, but it was something of a shock to the system to experience the threatening undercurrent of the attitude of some where the medical building was situated in not the most pleasant looking of places to say the least.

Most people seemed to notice us, and some stared menacingly as we walked by.

'Put your hair under your hat,' Ethan said, 'and don't look at anyone; just focus on where we are going.'

We were approached a few times by aggressive people, and I felt unnerved by the area, but Ethan reasoned, 'This may be the only place that can treat you because of the type of cancer you have. You might be safe in the actual building.'

There were some nice-seeming people in the area of course and some said hello to me while I sat in the waiting room for my appointment and I would reciprocate in greeting them with politeness, but generally most others just gawped at me, as though they could not believe what they were seeing, or loudly demanded that I talk to them, behaviour that I had no choice but to put up with until I was called in to see the surgeon.

'Your particular type of cancer's treatment requires careful planning,' my assigned lead surgeon, a very courteous woman, explained to me when I met her at the appointment. 'You have a high-grade adenocarcinoma, a rarer kind of cervical cancer. It is situated deep in the cervix and is an anterior tumour, growing towards the bladder.'

I listened calmly to everything she told me and remained so as she explained that this type of tumour does not respond well, if at all, to chemotherapy, and that the only way to stop it in its tracks was to surgically remove it, along with any surrounding tissue and organs to prevent metastasis (spread of the cancer).

'These are the margins around your tumour,' said the surgeon, drawing a rough diagram of my reproductive system and its surrounding areas. 'Sometimes, in tumour surgery, they take this area'—she indicated the area surrounding my uterus on the diagram— 'but because your cancer is high-grade and can spread easily, it is imperative that we take this area away.' She drew a larger area that included tissues and many lymphatic nodes in the groin and up towards the bladder, as well as other parts of the pelvic area. 'I want to be absolutely sure that I take away any area that poses a considerable risk of metastasis. Also, because of the scale and length of the surgery, I will not be able to perform it alone, so there will be another surgeon present, and we will also be employing a new robotic technique.'

I stared at the diagram as I tried to take it all in. I knew that I was facing a huge surgery, and I knew that the surgery would result in the loss of some of my organs. The surgeon discussed with me the fact that I had never had children and how the treatment would leave me without a reproductive system.

A couple of weeks later, I received a letter that explained the results of the multi-disciplinary team discussion regarding the way forward with my treatment. There had been some deliberation over the options for this, since it was an unusual case. The Royal Marsden oncologist wanted to perform trachelectomy—the removal of the cervix—followed by aggressive courses of radiotherapy: he felt that the semi-exenterated surgery was too risky and felt that it could leave me with permanent significant health issues. The surgeon I had met with, meanwhile, felt that radiotherapy would have little to no effect on residual cancer cells of my type of tumour, and that large margins were necessary. While another specialist advised that even more of the abdominal area be removed, given the danger of this particular type of cancer spreading. All of their opinions were invaluable to me.

Discussions of this nature continued amongst the medical professionals for a couple of months as they debated among themselves which was the best route to take with my treatment and if they should venture into the more unknown techniques.

Then I was sent to see the female surgeon again, during which she seemed to be rather optimistic. 'I have a date for you in a few weeks' time for the surgery,' she said brightly.

Whilst I was incredibly grateful for such efficient plans for my treatment to have been arranged, I was daunted at the thought of having the surgery at the location in which it would take place, since it seemed to be a dangerous and extremely depressing area that Ethan and I were completely unfamiliar with and neither of us knew anyone there.

The surgeon explained, 'We have to get this cancer out of you! Radiotherapy will not get rid of your type of cancer, and neither will chemotherapy; we have to properly cut it out. Due to its high-grade nature, the cancer and any chance of its metastasising further needs to be stopped straight away.'

I knew the incredible seriousness of the situation and I realised that this was the only way forward. All things considered, the way to survive the cancer would be to tackle it radically—and this was the only place in which that could properly be done. So, I accepted it and was thankful.

The surgeon broached the subject of another aspect of my unusual case: oncological and surgical clinical research, and how I was a perfect candidate for this. It was explained that not enough was known about how to efficiently treat this type of gynae cancer—being as it was a high-grade cervical adenoma—particularly in young women, and so I was told that my case could be used in vital medical research and could help make important changes.

I thanked the surgeon for her time and assistance and was then sent to the support person who had been assigned to oversee my care.

She spoke of the emotional and practical aspects of the life-changing treatment that I was about to endure

'I don't know how I will get home after the surgery,' I told her, especially given that I lived quite far away from the area and Ethan did not drive.

'We will arrange for an ambulance to take you back,' reassured the support person.

It was mentioned that my particular case was valuable to oncological clinical research.

I left that appointment resigned to the fact that I had to accept the unnerving location of my treatment, despite confiding in the assigned nursing support person my feelings of great unease at the location of the building and my fears surrounding having my treatment there, given the disturbing behaviour that was so apparent in the area.

Though I was notably still filled with gratitude towards the surgeon and the healthcare available to me, the prospect of being alone in such a dangerous place when I was so unwell was nonetheless most unnerving.

The Royal Marsden was no longer an option, as it had been explained that the treatment that they proposed in my case, might not be as effective in the long-term as that which was available to me at the other establishment.

Therefore, it was agreed that in a few weeks' time, I would be undergoing life-changing surgery.

Though I of course felt fear about what I was about to undergo, I was completely calm and collected during this time. However, some people who had never had cancer told me that they would 'fight' cancer if they had it and 'not be all quiet like you are'. *What would they do,* I logically wondered, *fight their own body? Run around frantically fighting themselves?!* There was no fight to engage in, so far as I was concerned; just a need to restore the balance of healthy cells, and, with the aid of conventional medicine, I felt this to be entirely possible.

The talk of 'fighting' in relation to cancer, that is so expected these days, can be I feel, in the most respectful way, nonsensical and unhelpful. My perspective is that it is actually the treatment and the immune system that does the fighting (I say this with two points in mind: firstly, if we take the view that we should be seen to be 'fighting' the illness, then by that reckoning does that mean that someone who has sadly lost their life to cancer had not 'fought' enough? We know that not to be the case at all, especially when someone has been courageous in dealing with their illness. Secondly, the expectation to be seen to be 'fighting' the illness can place a burden on the ill person, when realistically, they may not feel like putting on a brave face consistently at this incredibly challenging time). The evidence-based medicine does its thing in combating the cancer. Meanwhile, the ill person reserves the physical strength and energy that their body so needs at this time, enjoying things that they like to do in life whenever they can. In this way, the situation can feel less daunting and frightening.

I continued with my focused approach and where I could, I also managed to continue with bouts of exercise as I knew that apart from the cancer, my body was still physically strong.

But the enormity of what I was about to undergo was still a frightening prospect. I knew that I would be alone; that Ethan would be alone and that he had nowhere safe to stay in the area where we would be; that he knew nobody there; that I may be unsafe at the building where my surgery would take place; that the surgery was going to severely damage my body forever; that there was a very good chance that I might not survive the surgery at all.

And yet, I felt that I could get through it. I was completely serene in facing my fear.

8
The Trepidation of a Dignified Shield Maiden

WINTER WAS NOW BEGINNING, AND the day of the life-changing radical surgery arrived.

My main concern was for Ethan: I had always tried to look out for him and his health and happiness every day ever since we had first got together and now, I worried for his wellbeing whilst I was undergoing the surgery and not able to help him while I was recovering from it, and even more so if I did not survive it. He had always been an immensely capable and extremely resilient guy, but he had been through some incredibly tough times throughout his life, and I didn't want him to suffer further.

Although fearful at my own imminent circumstances, the practicalities of my situation took precedence. There seemed to be endless practical issues to attend to under the circumstances, and there was no time, no room, no place, for getting upset.

The dreaded day of the life-changing medical treatment came, and that late afternoon, as I looked around at the building where the surgery was due to take place, with thugs hanging around outside and knowing the enormity of what I was about to go through, I felt fear.

From my life experience, when we are truly in an extremely serious and threatening situation, we typically will not cry immediately: the weeping due to an outpouring of emotion comes later, usually after the event, when the mind attempts to process the complex emotions related to what has just been witnessed or suffered. In the actual moment of the experience, however, it seems that we subconsciously focus on the fight-or-flight process. I knew that here, 'flight' was not an option—that would mean the cancer being allowed to rapidly metastasize—and so that left me with no option but to face this head-on.

I felt a rather simple acceptance at this point: I had no option but to endure this. For all of my life, some mistakenly viewed my gentleness as weakness, completely underestimating what lay beneath that: an understanding and ability of how to, for the most part, adapt and endure, even when alone and in dire circumstances.

So, here I was, sitting on the clinical bed allocated to me in the vast, long, old room that contained many other beds. Ethan and I had been immediately surprised at the very little order in place and the large number of visitors there, who were the cause of much noise and chaos. Some of the nurses had decided to put me in the first bed by the entrance, an area where everyone could see me, rather than in the separate rooms for seriously ill people, where I would have perhaps been safer. I felt anxious at the complete lack of privacy and being amongst all the chaos but of course grateful for being provided with a medical bed and treatment.

We were also surprised to find that I was one of only two cancer patients, and that most of the other patients were only there for minor issues; a mishmash with no particular speciality, which is quite irregular.

A lovely nurse called Gina came to me to check me in as a patient. She studied me thoughtfully while attaching a patient identity band to my wrist and progressing through the routine questions and checks.

She smilingly complimented me and added 'You are different to the people I usually meet!' These comments were kind, and I appreciated the friendly sentiment to them, but they reinforced my self-consciousness that I was standing out—and standing-out here, in this kind of unruly environment, was not safe.

Ethan left me with Gina while he went to make a phone call. When he returned, he told me, 'I was just nearly mugged downstairs. I'm fine, but I reported it to the security, and they said that it happens all the time!'

As my surgery was extensive and required two surgeons, the

other surgeon, who I had not met before, came to speak to me. She was an enthusiastic and chatty woman in her late thirties, and she spoke to me about the surgery and what both surgeons had planned. She explained the possible risks and outcomes before then going on to discuss the ongoing research in that area of medicine at that time, and how they would like to film the surgery, with my consent, since my case was unusual. She seemed very enthusiastic to get the chance to practice on me, telling me that opportunities like this were scarce; not only was my case of cancer quite unusual, I was told, but my body was also naturally in as good a shape as could be. Throw in the fact that I had never had any children and was a physically fit and lithe young woman, and we apparently had a rare combination indeed—things that were all very good news for this element of surgical and cancer research.

Before providing my consent, I considered that this would all be very intrusive on my privacy and, for that matter, my dignity. Saying this, such pioneering research could help to prevent so many young women from suffering from some of the same pain that I had—and so, for the second time in my life, I forwent my privacy and allowed the intrusion of clinical research into my body and circumstances to help advance female oncological medicine.

The first time I had done so had been several years earlier, when I was diagnosed with a benign breast tumour (I would go on to develop several of them and just learn to live with them). Though painful, it was completely harmless. To me, a 'scare', as that benign breast tumour was, is a nothingness: there is no drama, and we are not ill. Rather than such an experience being upsetting, it should simply make us feel extra grateful of good health. That is how I felt about it and, though I would live with the tumour, I gratefully got on with my life and immediately put the whole episode behind me. However, I had been approached by a Consultant Scientist and some of his staff who had been very keen to enrol me on a new medical study and asked me to help, stating that the combination of the benign tumour, my biometrics and fitness levels made me a good prospect for the study. He told me that the research he was doing could be vital to developing understanding of the causes of breast cancer. I had been a little taken aback when they told me that it was a new study and that I would be in the first few; 'nothing like this has been done before, and there would be nothing in it for you as the contributor. We would need samples of your bloodwork and of your benign tumour, and to monitor you every now and then for the rest of your life—but it *would* be very helpful', he had explained. After learning that there was a possibility that this study could prevent some women from developing breast cancer, it felt natural that it was my duty, in a sense, to contribute my help and so I agreed to being part of their research. Little did I know then that I had become a tiny initial part of a hugely significant, ground-breaking part of history that would go on to discover the BRCA gene—the cause of some breast cancers. Indeed, the work of the brilliant consultants and the research team would go on to save many lives all over the world.

Well, before, with the clinical research that I was involved with in my ongoing participation with the Breakthrough cancer study, I had been but a minute cog in a machine; but now, with this high-grade cervical cancer I found myself to be something of an integral part of another cancer research entity, and the experience was far more invasive to say the least.

Though I was troubled by maintaining my dignity as part of the clinical research,, I knew that I had to put any of my own thoughts and feelings to one side however: this, after all, was about people's lives, for my fellow females and their loved ones; to aid in advancement of gynaecological cancer treatment and so I gave my consent to help.

The surgery, in my unusual case, would be filmed clinically and the film used to train surgeons developing new techniques, therefore preventing many young women from going through the extent of what I endured.

After the visit from the surgeon and they had left, it suddenly began to get even busier and louder in the very long room—most unusually loud for a medical building, by anyone's reckoning. An array of noises filled the space: shouting; alarms; chairs being dragged across the floor; loud chatting on mobile phones; sinister laughing; arguing. It suddenly struck me that there seemed to be no rules, no order. I was also unnerved to overhear some of the visitors loudly discussing things pertaining to obtaining narcotics, what place had been "done over", who had been arrested, who they had threatened, what stolen goods they knew someone had available...

Some of the people could not seem to believe what they were seeing in my being there—something that Ethan and a couple of the nurses commented on, saying that I was standing out. I tried, despite my unease and fear, to be friendly and polite to them and when they approached my bedspace, but then again, remaining courteous after being subjected to abusive comments right when you have cancer and are preparing to undergo a massive surgery that has a good chance of killing you or affecting you for life is challenging. There were some nice people there too, of course, but the disturbing behaviour of some of those present made me just want to flee the place.

The time came for Ethan to leave. I was terribly worried about him. We had very little money and so consequently nowhere nearby or decent for him to stay for the following weeks. his only option under the circumstances, over five miles away, a squalid building, where he had to sleep on the floor among some cushions and with a sleeping bag. I would only later learn how very cold and uncomfortable this had been for him, as at the time, he did not tell me the extent of how bad his own circumstances were, perhaps not wanting me to stress over them.

He politely tried to ask a nurse that as I was having radical surgery for cancer treatment early the next day and the odds were that I might not survive, could he please see me in the morning? She told him that he could not, insisting that I should have instead been treated in the area in which I lived and that she didn't think it was right that I was using their services.

I tried to gently explain that I had been referred here due to the particular skill and specialized equipment needed to treat my case of cancer; that the surgeons had been very eager to have me as a patient, and that I was very grateful for the treatment, but they further commented, 'well, you've got yourself into this situation anyway'. I wondered what they meant by that.

To say that I was extremely uneasy about the environment that I was in would not be doing the grimness of this reality justice. Regardless, I knew that I had to get through it.

I suddenly felt more vulnerable than ever: some of the rowdy patients and visitors stared intently at me, and as this felt intimidating, I tried to avoid all eye contact with them. With my bed standing directly at the entrance to the ward, there was a handbasin right next to me, and it seemed that every few minutes, somebody—usually a man—was coming to use this facility. Being directly next to the handbasin, along with the entrance to the room, meant that there was zero privacy in the bedspace.

'I've never seen so many visitors washing their hands,' said Gina when we were interrupted again as she returned to do more of my paperwork and health checks to get me settled in.

She seemed to latch onto what was going on. 'Hmm, actually, this isn't the best place to have put you. I had no say in that, but I'll see what I can do.'

I tried to cope with the unruly and intimidating behaviour that I was surrounded by as best I could, but it grew worse. Ultimately, I fled to the far end of the room in an attempt to get away from the unbearable racket and chaos. I bumped into Gina, who was coming out of the TV room.

'Gina, I'm sorry but I can't stand it here,' I tearfully explained. 'I can cope with my cancer, but not this; all the noise and crazy behaviour.'

After telling her what I had seen and what had been said, Gina took me into the TV room with her arm around me, trying to console me. 'I know what you mean, Rebecka; I work here, and this is what we have to put up with most of the time. People think we get used to it as nurses, but we don't.'

'Oh, Rebecka,' said another lovely nurse, overhearing the conversation, and taking hold of my hand in comfort. 'It drives us mad, too!'

'I have never witnessed anything like this in a medical establishment,' I said quietly. 'Is it going to be like this all the time?'

The answer was pretty much that nothing could be done about the situation. The nurses looked at me helplessly and told me that they understood. We chatted for a little while about nice things, trying to take our minds off what was going on outside the room. The nurses meant it when they said that they would try to help me as best as they could but told me that both would not be at work for the majority of my stay. The lovely nurses then had to return to their duties, and Gina took me back to my bed.

Visiting time was now over, and yet there were still men there who continued in their staring at me as I walked past them and across the long room. Although it was late in the evening by now and the other patients were getting ready for bed, I did not feel safe changing into my nightdress while the male visitors were there and almost watching my every move.

But I was most concerned about Ethan. He is an incredibly tough man, but his injuries as a result of his military service could be painful at times. The thought of him being alone, with no access to any comforts, and having nobody to look out for him, as I usually did, in a completely unfamiliar area and one such as this in particular, walking back very late at night during an incredibly harsh, bitterly icy winter, distressed me and I worried terribly for his wellbeing and safety.

Eventually, all the visitors left. Gina and the other lovely nurse had both gone home, but one of the night nurses was kind to me.

I was exhausted: my whole body and mind was not only dealing with the imminent surgery, the tumour, and all of my worries, but my stress hormones and adrenaline had surged at a constant level for many hours because of everything going on around me, and I now felt tired. But I couldn't allow myself to try and sleep until around the time that Ethan would hopefully have made it back safely to where he was staying.

The huge room was now much quieter, although I could hear shouting and violence outside. I lay down with my worries and fears still whirring around my mind, and thought with a heavy heart, *I might not survive tomorrow, and I have never been able to achieve anything truly meaningful in my life because each time I tried or had the opportunity to, I was either ill or prevented from doing so. My life has been a waste.*

At some point during the night, I managed to fall asleep. My life would, in just a few hours, never be the same again.

Early in the morning, for comfort at what I was about to endure, I had wanted to see some of the nature I had found endless solitude in all my life, but upon looking outside the bathroom window, I saw nothing but dreary grey office-style buildings, and a car park. No greenery; no nature; not even a tree. It was truly a depressing scene.

Disheartened, I changed into the surgical gown, as instructed, and managed to stay very calm. I had a great deal of faith that I could survive the surgery, as I knew that I had prepared my body well with my healthy lifestyle, and with what I knew from having had some physiology training.

Given that the nurses would not allow Ethan to see me, he called just before I was taken down to theatre, but a nurse told me off for using the phone at the nurse's station to answer his call, though the other patients were allowed to do so freely. When I gently explained the importance of the phone call, given what I was about to go through with the treatment for cancer, they simply sarcastically replied, 'so?'.

Ethan told me that although the surgery would take place all day, he would come to the building in the morning, just in case he was needed and even though he had to wait outside.

The thought of him sitting alone the entire day, made me feel sad.

But I tried to remain calm and composed as one of the theatre team, a young guy, came to collect me to take me to theatre, pushing me some distance in the hospital bed.

Yes, there was a good chance that I would not survive this radical surgery, with its partly pioneering techniques, but instead, I chose to focus on there also being a chance that I would. I simply felt, *my body has got this: It's in control.*

The theatre team, complete with two surgeons, were very keen to get straight into the surgery, as it would take all day, so I was quickly prepped in a bay adjacent to the theatre. I was not allowed to see the theatre itself, as it was full of robotic equipment and lots of staff. I felt fear at this point, but I remained calm.

The lead surgeon came over and said hello warmly. As the anaesthetist prepared to put me under, two kind and caring male theatre nurses stood on either side of me. One was middle-aged with a gentle voice, while the other was the young guy who had taken me down to theatre.

'I'm scared,' I told them softly.

They each held one of my hands affectionately. I felt truly, absolutely safe with them and incredibly fortunate to have such conscientious professionals looking after me.

'Just imagine yourself on a tropical beach, with the sea and the sunshine and the palm trees, listening to the waves on the sand, feeling peaceful,' said the elder male theatre nurse as the anaesthetist placed the mask over my nose and mouth. 'Beautiful beach, relaxing on the sand, palm trees. Peaceful...'

9
Survival

'REBECKA. REBECKA.'
THE FIRST THING I heard was a muffled female voice, accompanied by a tapping on the face and hand and quickly followed by the beeping of medical machinery.

'Rebecka. Can you hear me?'

'Rebecka, wake up.'

'Still not responding.'

Beep. Beep. Beep. Beep.

I could hear the voices and the noises, but they sounded faded, like they were coming from somewhere far away. It took a few moments for them to become clearer.

Beep. Beep. Beep.

'Rebecka, can you hear me?'

Yes, I can hear you, I thought very hazily.

'Rebecka, wake up.'

I must have lightly opened my eyes.

'Ahh, she's with us.'

'Rebecka, the surgery is over now.'

'We're glad to have you back with us. We've been trying to wake you for ages,' said a friendly male voice.

With an oxygen mask over my face and a dense, heavy feeling that strangely felt like having been hit over the head with something, I could barely mumble or open my eyes. I was extremely unwell indeed—more ill and immobile than I could ever have imagined in my wildest dreams. I had been unresponsive for some time, it transpired, and the theatre team had worked hard doing their amazing job in stabilizing me, therefore keeping me alive.

I can barely recall what was said or what happened next and could hardly keep my eyes open—but sometime later, I was wheeled on the medical bed with the oxygen attached, through the corridors.

I suddenly heard Ethan's voice. 'Is she okay? She looks so pale,' he said to one of the theatre nurses.

'She's been through a rough time; that amount of surgery was a bit of a shock to her body' they replied gently. 'We were concerned for a while, but she's stable now. We need to keep a close eye on her, though.'

'Beck, it's me,' said Ethan, grasping my hand as he walked alongside the theatre nurses who were pushing my bed through the vast corridors of the building and back to my bedspace in the very long, chaotic room. 'Can you open your eyes, Beck? Can you squeeze my hand?'

I think I did, but that was all the movement that I could manage: I felt paralysed and nauseous. I just wanted to sleep.

'She looks so angelic even though she's been through all of that,' a nurse said to Ethan. He apparently thought so too and told me that some others had continued to comment in this manner, though I cannot imagine that I looked anything other than like the dreadfully ill person that I was at the time. But strangely, being seen in this way was why I was about to attract a great deal of completely unwanted attention at my most ultimately vulnerable.

I can hardly remember any of the rest of the evening as I drifted in and out of sleep, unable to talk or move. I was attached to a number of drips and tubes, including one for morphine, but I could not feel any of them at this stage.

One of the surgeons and the anaesthetist popped in at one point to talk to Ethan, but I don't recall anything that they said to each other apart from them saying that the treatment part of the surgery had gone well. In a post-anaesthetic and heavily morphine-induced stupor, I must have been fairly unconscious until midday the next day.

'Rebecka,' said a nurse as I opened my eyes slowly, 'we think you might have stabilised enough to remove the oxygen now. Let's see if we can get you up.'

The oxygen mask was removed, and another nurse helped to lift my delicate frame and move me out of bed in order to give me a bed bath and change the bed sheets. Pain seared through my pelvic and abdominal area, despite the morphine being pumped through my body, and I struggled to keep my eyes open. My disorientation remained, and the room spun. I could hardly speak and felt sort of almost paralysed.

I was completely consumed by the feeling of being so terribly, horribly unwell.

The nurses carefully manoeuvred the drips and tubes that I was attached to, placing my feet over the edge of the bed, and their arms beneath mine, getting me onto the chair at my bedside. I suddenly became aware of the Foley catheter that was attached to me via a bag by my bed.

Nausea overcame me as I was brought to my feet by the nurses, and I was suddenly more unwell in that regard than I ever thought it possible to be.

In my severe state of physical weakness, I trembled uncontrollably and whimpered in agony. The room had felt as though it was spinning the moment the nurses had gotten me out of bed. The immense dizziness that I felt became too much and it seemed that I had sort of fainted as the nurses placed me on the chair. I opened my eyes to find them rushing around me, taking my blood pressure and checking on all of the machines, drips, and tubes.

'It's okay,' one of them said. 'That's to be expected after such large surgery.'

The nurses left me on the chair while the bedsheets were changed, then bringing a bowl of water and a cloth to give me a bed bath as best as they could. My long hair had been kept in a plait for the last couple of days, and it tumbled over my shoulder.

My body was trying to adjust to the enormity of what it had just been through, and I was acutely unwell. I was about as vulnerable as it is possible to be.

The nurses were busy with lots of tasks to complete, and as they went off to do other things, left me in the chair. The room was becoming noisier as visitors piled in, and there were men regularly using the handbasin at the side of my bed. I felt uneasy at this, but it hardly registered, as I could not stop myself from falling asleep in my heavily post-surgical state.

I opened my eyes to find two scruffy-looking men standing by my bed, staring directly at me. Startled, I made some kind of muffled yelping sound in my physical weakness. I heard the nurses' voices coming closer to my bedspace as they spoke to them, and the men quickly went.

Feeling so ill and incapable of a response, I simply trembled. The fear lessened gradually, however, and I fell back to sleep, the effects of the anaesthetic once again overcoming me. I quickly heard chatter and shouting again but did not open my eyes. There had also been an alarm that made a clattering sound going off throughout the morning by the opposite side of the entrance, and I was trying to block out the din.

Then, in amongst all the chaos, I heard Ethan's voice: 'Beck, what are you doing there, out of bed?'

I had not noticed through my pain and disorientation that I was almost on the floor, half-naked and with the various attached tubes in disarray.

He searched for a nurse and told them how he had found me almost on the floor. They blamed the junior nurse for that, even though she had been sent to work elsewhere for most of the morning. I winced with pain as Ethan and a nurse put me back into bed, still in a sitting-upright position. Ethan became aware of the room filling up with visitors who were once again gawping at me. He wanted to pull the curtains around my bed to protect my dignity, but the nurses would not let him do so.

'I don't mean to bother you, but people are staring at her all the time. She's attracting attention, and it's not safe,' he said. 'Other patients who are in here for minor things are allowed to have the curtains around their bed, especially at visiting times.'

'Well, *she* can't,' said the nurse sternly, referring to me in a hateful tone.

He did as he was told, and the staring and deliberate walking past my bed continued.

If I had been a spectacle before, now, I was an exhibition.

It was very noisy in the room again. I was in a great deal of pain and unable to move, sitting completely upright, possibly being that the elevation helped some part of the post-surgical recovery. Ethan was then sharply told to leave, despite the fact that there were other male visitors still sitting around the beds.

'She shouldn't even be here, using our services. You should have gone to your own area,' they told him.

'But you let in all of the other male visitors all day long, even the aggressive and disruptive ones,' he quietly explained in confusion.

'They're locals!' the nurse snapped at him.

The angry nurses didn't care about all the male visitors coming in and out of the room. Strangely, they would angrily prevent Ethan—who was polite and helpful and whom some of the nurses liked talking to—from being in the room, but not the aggressive, disruptive visitors.

I felt a strong urge to just sleep; I so wanted to lie down and sleep off the effects of the massive surgery but with my bed being in that raised up high sitting position I couldn't. My body was devoid of any strength, and I was still struggling to even keep my eyes open. However, actual sleep was almost impossible due to the noise level in the large lengthy room, and so I just sat there, mentally managing the noise and the pain and the detached feeling of *is this really happening?*

Some time passed before I finally drifted off, when I suddenly awoke with a start: there was a man who I had never seen before standing by my bed. He was observing me eagerly. He began to move closer to me, standing by my feet and raising his hand, as if, it seemed, he was going to touch me.

This moment must have only lasted a few seconds, but it felt like longer. I tried to shout out for someone to come to my rescue, but because of my very ill post-surgical state and the morphine I'd been administered, the sound that came out was more like a yelp.

It seemed, however, that this was enough: the man quickly headed out of the ward entrance. A nurse came to check on me, as I trembled with fear.

'What's the matter, Rebecka?' asked a flustered-looking nurse.

'There was a man,' I mumbled. 'Please move me out of here,' I begged faintly.

The nurse looked for the man, but he had left. 'But he didn't touch you?' she asked.

'No,' I whimpered.

The nurse assumed that the man must have simply got the wrong patient by mistake.

The lead surgeon came to check on me and told Ethan that it was going to be a very long recovery.

Gina walked in. She smiled and waved at me as she walked past my bed. It was comforting to see her.

Then, before I knew it, it was early evening and visiting time again. There was a lovely family who visited throughout the day to see a young woman on the opposite side of the room a few beds down who had also undergone surgery, and they seemed to be really caring people, and were the quietest and most respectful there. They always waved to me and smiled warmly when they walked past my bed, looking concerned. Such civilised behaviour, however, was unfortunately an absolute rarity in this building.

Slowly but surely, more visitors than I had ever seen so far began to pile into the room, and the tumultuous racket was becoming unbearable. Most didn't talk but shouted, sometimes from one end of the room to the other.

Every few minutes, it seemed some man was using the handbasin by my bed, and they always stared straight at me like they could not believe what they were seeing. There were families gathered around the beds of the patients opposite to me, some just sitting and watching me and even having a discussion over the way I looked. Not all of them were so aggressive or nosey, but most of them seemed to have no sense of social boundaries, politeness, or even any awareness of seriously ill people's suffering.

When Ethan walked in, I could tell he was shocked by what he saw: strangers gawping at me and standing near my bed. He told them off. Gina walked back in, having left earlier to attend to tasks. She was similarly unsettled by the scene and came to me straight away.

'Are you okay, Rebecka?' she asked me.

I could open my eyes more now and speak a little, and so I

managed to tell her how frightened I was, how ill I felt, and how unbearable the noise was. She looked deeply concerned.

'Can we get her moved?' pleaded Ethan. 'It's not safe for her here. She shouldn't be under threat at a time like this.'

'I know... I'm very concerned about her, but I'm limited with what I can do,' she responded empathetically, 'We can't stop the visitors coming in, and if they are only staring at her or standing by her bedside, security can't do anything. This certainly wasn't the best place to put her.'

I felt so desperately ill. The loud, persistent chatter; the obnoxious, repetitive shouting; the cackling laughter; the loud alarm at the entrance constantly ringing; the staring, like I was a creature in a zoo. With my bed raised to its highest so that I was fully sitting up, and, with the curtains fully pulled back around it, all I could see was the many staring faces gathered around the beds, looking back at me. I was overwhelmed by this excruciating torment that taunted my senses so soon after receiving radical, life-changing surgery for treatment of cancer, lying there with my wounds and drips and tubes and catheter bag, overcome by pain to an intensity that I never thought possible. *Make it go away. Please* make it stop, *make it stop.* The noise, the staring, the pain, the people loitering around my bed, the complete and utter mayhem... I could not withstand this any longer.

My eyes were open, and I was as alert as I could be as the distress started to take acutely hold of me. I could take no more. I began to try to move. I just wanted to get out, but of course, I could not do so: the surgery and morphine had rendered me almost immobile. I moved my arms in some motion, trying to get up out of bed and, in doing so, knocked a piece of medical equipment over, which made a loud crashing sound. *Make it stop. Please. Get me out of this place.*

Gina must have heard the noise, and she came rushing to me. 'Oh, Rebecka. Sweetheart...' She seemed distressed as she watched me attempting to move around and get out of bed and my pleading to leave. The machines that I was attached to were bleeping as my heart rate quickened. Gina pulled the curtains around my bed and took my blood pressure and temperature, which she told Ethan had both spiked, and said how helpless she felt: those in charge, it seemed, would not agree to her requests to move me or to inform the doctors of what I was going through.

Completely helpless, I was trapped in this crazy environment.

'*Please* get me out of here,' I begged. '*Please*. Get these people away from me. The noise. The shouting. The alarm... Please, I can't take anymore.'

'I know, I know, darling; I hear that alarm in my sleep,' said Gina wearily.

'Please get me out of here,' I cried and pleaded.

'Can we please move her somewhere safer and quieter?' Ethan insisted. 'There are more private areas where she would be much safer.'

'I really want to: that would be the best thing to do. But my hands are tied', said Gina, as she sat with me, her face most expressive of worry, explaining that I needed to lay still to get my heart rate and blood pressure to a safer level. My newly surgically shocked body was reacting dangerously to this threatening and torturous-to-the-senses situation. Gina held my hand, and Ethan held the other.

'How long is she going to have to be here?' Ethan asked Gina.

'How long is a piece of string?' she shrugged. 'She's very ill, and my requests to have her moved have been refused. She could be here for a while.'

They both regarded me with expressions of deep concern.

'Can we at least get the security to warn the visitors who approach her to leave her alone?' asked Ethan quietly, not wanting to get Gina into trouble.

She whispered back that there was a problem with the threatening behaviour of some visitors but were reluctant to doing anything about it as it could be seen as victimisation toward them. It was very apparent that this lovely and incredibly caring and efficient young nurse, who was brilliant at her job, was under great strain in her working conditions. Sadly, she did not seem to be the only one.

'These must be tough circumstances for you to be working in,' he said, and she quietly answered that she did, indeed, feel under a lot of stress at work. She told Ethan that today would be her last shift at work for a week, and that she would leave notes for the next shift of nurses detailing her recommendations for my care, including that I needed to be moved imminently to a safer and quieter area.

The clangour of the alarm, near the door and not far from my bedspace, continued, and Ethan asked Gina if something could be done about it. 'That would drive anyone mad, let alone a cancer patient who's just had massive surgery', he said.

Gina said that maintenance had been called to fix it to stop it going off repeatedly, but were unable to for a while, so there was nothing that could be done until then.

The visitors continued shouting and pretending to use the handbasin, and one pulled open the bed curtains that Gina had temporarily closed while she examined me. Ethan and Gina glared at him. Gina told me that she would make me as comfortable as she possibly could and confided to Ethan, 'She'll be on my mind now for days.'

After stabilising me, Gina returned to her duties and Ethan sat with me, holding my hand, while I continued whimpering for all of it to stop.

The visiting time eventually came to an end, and Ethan was told to leave. 'If anyone tries to touch you, you scream, okay?' instructed Ethan as he was leaving.

Exhausted, my whole mind and body in an acute state of stress, I could hardly respond. Gina came to see me before she left for a few days leave. She leaned over and embraced me affectionately. 'I've done the best I can for you,' she said quietly. 'I have made the necessary recommendations and urged that you're moved. I will be calling tomorrow to see if it's been done. I'll be thinking of you.' She left looking very stressed.

That night, there were still a couple of male visitors coming in and out of the room. However, the other visitors had gone, the alarm had been quietened temporarily, and as deep night fell, I managed to finally get a little sleep until tests were taken at my bedside, my blood tests and blood pressure readings still being abnormal.

After this was done and being awake, I overheard a couple of the staff discussing me. As well as discussing the way that I spoke (strangely, my not having a regional accent seemed to be an issue to them), they added commentary on the hideous situation that I had ended up in.

'It's her own fault she's like that, silly girl; that's what happens when you don't go for your smear tests.'

They had simply assumed the latter on the basis of my having cervical cancer and were totally ignorant of the fact that I had attended for all of my screening tests, always right on schedule and never missing any.

The searing, agonising post-surgical pain continued. There was occasionally a lovely nurse at night who came to me at this time. 'You press the control for your morphine, sweetheart. Keep topping it up as much as you need.'

In the morning, a doctor came to see me, checking my wounds and reading through the clinical notes at the foot of my bed, noting any abnormal observations. There was little that could be done at this stage except to monitor my recovery.

That alarm by the entrance started up again at full volume. I heard the nurses say something about the maintenance people coming to fix it, and, again, towards midday, the vast room filled with visitors once more.

One of the nurses, Fiona, a friendly girl, pulled the curtains around my bed and gently lifted me out of it, being mindful of the tubing and equipment attached to me, and put me on the chair while they changed the bed sheets. Male visitors regularly came to wash their hands at the washbasin again—some genuinely, of course, but generally, many were not even washing them; just gawping. There were other available washbasins, but they kept coming to use the one by my bedspace.

And then, just when I thought my dignity could not be any more invaded, as Fiona went to attend to something else, I sat topless on the chair, having just had a bed bath, a blanket covering my lower body. I looked up to see a man looking through the curtains at my bare breasts, with an expression of lecherous abandon. He caught the eye of the other nurse—and her only reaction was to pull the curtain properly around.

It was shortly after this that Ethan came to see me, and I begged him to get me out of here. He politely spoke to the nurses about this again, to no avail: there was nothing they could do. One of the nurses snapped at Ethan, telling him to leave. He gently mentioned about the other male visitors being allowed into the room constantly. They had been very smug about this, openly mocking Ethan's suffering at being outside alone in the icy cold. 'They're locals', the nurse replied to Ethan.

A woman who was regularly visiting another female patient in the same room as me, had previously overheard that I had cervical cancer and listening to the nurses' conversation with him, added, 'It's your partners' own fault she's in that mess. She should have gone for her smear tests'. The two nurses who knew the visitor looked at Ethan with an expression of agreement at this comment. Ethan tried to explain that I had actually attended for all of my cervical screening tests immediately and had never missed one, but they were having none of it; as far as they were concerned, that just wasn't possible as my cancer would have been picked up on the tests.

Later, the same visitor, as she was walking past my bed, stopped and looked straight at me as she sneered, 'you've brought your cancer on yourself. Serves you right for not going for your tests. You deserve what you've got. You shouldn't get any help'.

Ethan asked one of the nicer nurses again if something could be done about the faulty alarm—and, surprisingly, this time, within hours, the maintenance person arrived, and the drilling noise of the alarm was eventually stopped. The relief to the senses was instant.

A lovely nurse who had assisted me on the first day entered the room, returning my wave. 'Hello, darling,' she said warmly. I asked how she was, and she touched my hand, and I held hers in return. She, too, had that look of helplessness; of seeming to be restricted in terms of what she could do.

The night was fairly similar to the previous one, except, mercifully, for the noise of the alarm. The nurses once again openly discussed me and my apparent stupidity regarding my cervical screening tests and erroneous placement.

During the night, I became seriously uncomfortable due to my being completely sat upright the whole time. Sometimes, as it was explained to me, patients who have had such large surgery might have to be placed in this position for various reasons, one possibly being to alleviate pressure on the surgical area, but all that I wanted to do was lie down somewhere quiet and sleep and it was extremely uncomfortable to be sat completely upright the whole time. Throughout the night, although I struggled to feel any movement in my lower body, in my subconsciousness, I must have shuffled a little at a time down the bed, being desperate to lie down and sleep, because in the morning, having finally had a few hours relief from the noise and chaos of the room, I was awoken by the voice of a male doctor—and I became aware that I was lying in a heap at the foot end of the bed, with the tubes all over the place. The doctor was wondering what had happened and why I had been left that way. He fetched a friendly young nurse who I had not seen before. 'This is Meena', the doctor said, 'she is going to look after you.'

Meena was a cheerful ball of energy. 'Hello! Let's get you sorted out.' She gently helped me out of bed and supported me as I stood, still attached to the drips and the Foley catheter, and linked me with her arm. She was patient and kind as I took my first tentative steps away from the bed. We walked very slowly down the vast room—a strange feeling, since I found that I could not feel the floor under my feet properly.

There were hardly any visitors during the early mornings when the doctors were present, so I was not being gawped at right now. It took us some time to reach the bathroom, and, just as we got there, another nurse called for Meena to attend to something urgently. With that, Meena left me with one of the not-so-nice staff, believing that I would be in safe hands, as she gave her instructions for my care.

'Come on, you can see to things yourself. There's the bathroom,' the nurse said shortly, ushering me into the tiny, enclosed, stuffy, windowless room. I watched her close the heavy door.

Just about managing to stand and still trembling from what my body had endured, with the drips, tubing, and catheter (and attached bag), and clinging onto the bathroom fittings for support and wondering how I was going to figure this out, I felt incredibly physically weak and the agonising pain from the surgery seared through me. This would also be my first time seeing how my body had been affected by the cancer treatment in the abdominal area and the surgical wounds.

I managed to juggle holding the drips, tubing, and bag enough to reach the seat in the shower, where I undressed with great difficulty, having to bring my nightdress over my head and carefully pass it over the IV tubing and bags. And then I looked down. I got a shock; my formerly flat and toned abdomen was very distended. And then there were several incredibly sore scars on my abdomen, naval and groin, covered in dressings. However, the talented surgeons had done such a brilliantly neat job that the scars would fade in time and the majority of the scarring was entirely internal, though more difficult and painful to heal.

But I told myself to get on with the situation. I managed to turn on the shower, avoiding the dressings as much as I could. I tried my best but, within minutes, the tiny room, poorly ventilated as it was, grew hotter—a stifling heat that overcame me. I turned off the shower with difficulty, my hand attached to a drip. I frantically pressed the alarm for the nurse, but nobody came. I tried again, in vain.

The room became hotter still. I cried out, 'Nurse, nurse...' No response.

I felt that at any minute, I would pass out, but I tried to compose myself. I pressed and pressed the alarm.

'Please! Help me,' I heard myself shout, pressing and pressing the alarm. I began to feel that I was starting to lose consciousness, and I slumped forward, trying to concentrate on my breathing, but it was getting too much. Everything went dark.

The next thing I knew, I opened my eyes to see Meena, fretting and asking me if I was alright. She had believed that she had left me in safe hands with the other nurse. She held the door open a little to let out the steam. She called for help and another nurse quickly arrived. They took my blood pressure and heart rate, which revealed that both had soared. Together, they got me dressed and lifted me out of the shower, placing their arms under mine.

I was later told that, in my heavily post-surgical and immobile state and with my body having just undergone such trauma, I should never have been left completely unsupervised in the bathroom. The nurse who had left me shot me a look of utter contempt as I walked past her and it would not be for the last time.

Ethan came to see me in the afternoon and found me being gawped at by visitors again, with some men standing staring near to my bed while I lay in agony, distressed at the staring.

Nothing could be done to protect me.

It was pure bad luck that all of this would keep happening, as the nurses who did look after me could, of course, only be there at certain times and I felt very sorry for them always being rushed off their feet. The rest of the time, I was entirely at the mercy of anyone's rage or twisted curiosity.

But the worst of this was yet to come.

10

Trapped

AT THIS POINT, THE NOISE levels were not quite as bad as the previous evenings: Meena, Fiona, and a couple of other nurses had ensured that there was more order and control being exercised within the room while they were there, and the alarm's volume had been minimised. The next rotation of staff came in, and during the last half an hour or so of talking to Ethan before he had to leave at the end of visiting hours, I had a strange feeling; a sensation that was like being on a waterbed.

After Ethan left, I wiggled around as much as I could, thinking that something did not feel right. I put my hand under the bedsheets. The bed felt soaking wet and, oddly, so did my back. I pulled the bedsheets back to find to my shock that the whole of the bed was soaked in a huge pool of... water? *No*, I thought, as the realisation dawned on me that the catheter could have leaked all over the bed.

'Excuse me,' I broached apprehensively to the first nurse to next walk past my bed. It was the first time I had asked any of the medical staff for help.

'What do you want? I'm busy,' she snapped.

'I'm sorry but I have a problem,' I said sheepishly, gesturing to the bed.

She looked angry at what she saw. 'You've wet the bed! How have you managed that?!'

'I don't know', I replied as I hung my head in shame and in quiet distress, 'I can't believe it. I feel so ashamed. I am so sorry. I'm sorry.'

The fluid, however, did not seem to be of that type. Plus, I had a catheter attached to the bladder.

But the nurse snapped, 'You *must* have known that you had; you *must* have known that you were lying in that! The bed's soaked.'

'But I couldn't feel it properly because of the effects of the morphine,' I sobbed. 'I am so sorry. I don't want to bother you.'

'You must have been messing with the catheter. Well, I can't do anything about it now; I'm busy. You'll have to wait. It's your *own* fault for not doing anything about it sooner,' she huffed.

An hour passed—and I was still lying in the soaked bed, in my soaked nightdress. I had never asked the staff for anything, but now, I felt so uncomfortable, lying in this condition, that I softly asked for their assistance.

'I'm sorry to bother you, but please could you—'

'No! You'll have to wait, you silly girl.'

Hours passed and as I lay there, I wondered had I managed to do this with a catheter attached. I already knew that the surgery had affected my bladder due to the position of the tumour—the surgeon had explained it to me—but I had not expected myself to do anything like this. I felt overcome by shame.

Then, the nurse appeared. 'Right, what have you been doing to the catheter?' she asked. 'That's completely bypassed the catheter. You've wet yourself.'

I looked at her with confusion and apologised profusely but added, 'I'm sorry but I haven't touched the catheter.'

She snapped again, 'You must have known that you were lying in that.'

'I'm sorry but I couldn't feel it,' I answered gently. 'It is difficult to feel much from the waist down because of the effects of the surgery and the morphine; it was only when it soaked my back that I became aware of it.'

She told her colleague that I had an incontinence problem. This apparent diagnosis was enough to reduce me to tears, as it was one of my worst fears realised.

'What's the matter, you silly girl?' the nurse snapped as she firmly placed her hands on my shoulders, giving them a light shake 'You are getting yourself upset again! The doctors can send you to psychiatry if you keep getting upset like this, and I might recommend that they do.' She spoke to me as though I was a misbehaved child rather than a quiet individual who behaved with deference towards them and who had just undergone huge physical trauma with cancer treatment in the worst of circumstances—and I felt just as helpless as a small child, too. But I continued to apologise profusely.

Being referred to as 'silly girl' in reference to being interpreted as a teenager because I looked so much younger than my age, was something that I had become used to.

Speaking would get me into trouble: every word could lead to me being referred to be forced into psychoanalysis—and in that moment, I truly realised that I had absolutely no control over what happened to me in any way; that I was at the complete mercy of others, be they the not-so-understanding nurses or the most sinister of the visitors; that I could not run; that I could hardly move at all.

Now, here, I was trapped in a solitary world of painful, degrading, overwhelming torment and fear from which there was no escape.

That night, the staff were openly discussing if they should tell the doctor, given that I had been previously assessed by a psychiatrist for 'psychosomatic' pain and bleeding due to 'possible depression', that they thought I should be referred back to the psychology department for 'crying and getting upset'. Hearing this terrified me.

Meanwhile, a young woman had been admitted in the night for a few hours, and her male visitors were coming in and out of the ward, with one standing near my bedspace and gawping lecherously across at me.

After he had gone, I ruminated over how I was going to face life with incontinence. The surgeon had previously told me that my bladder might possibly not return to function, and that another operation may be required to remove it and form a urostomy. *How was I going to tell Ethan*?, I wondered.

In the morning, assisted by one of the nurses, I got up to have a shower and the fluid leaked everywhere as I walked, a trail of it following my every step.

The fluid was not repellent in any way—it was an only very faintly coloured liquid, denser in consistency than water—but it was shocking to see the volumes of it of which flowed from me.

The nurse begrudgingly took me to a larger shower area this time but complained about how I was an inconvenience to them, being that most of the other patients there did not have immediate complex medical needs as a result of treatment and were there only for minor routine surgery.

'I am really trying to help myself. I do not want to bother anyone,' I told the nurse.

She did not respond and left me by the shower room door. This very dingy room was larger than the previous one that I had almost lost consciousness in.

I was still having trouble with feeling the ground beneath my feet. I lost my footing and slipped—and the next thing I knew, I was on the floor, with the tubes and drips attached and in agonising pain. I pressed the emergency buzzer, to which a very sweet and kind nurse responded by dashing in.

'Oh, lovey! Oh, dear! Are you okay?'

She could not have been any more helpful or conscientious. She gently helped me to stand up, checking my wounds and the tubing and helping me to dry and put my nightdress on. She seemed very concerned. 'Are you okay, Rebecka? You know, if you need to talk about anything, you can.'

I wanted to tell her the extent of what was happening to me but was too frightened to say anything about my experiences, fearing the consequences, and I also did not want the nice nurses to become involved in any kind of trouble, knowing that it was possible that some of their colleagues might make their working life more difficult, so I just looked at the floor while thanking her for her kindness. I think she knew some of what was happening to me, and yet I could not tell her: the fear was too great to speak out.

Regardless, both this nurse and Meena suspected that I was traumatised in some way, too wise with their instinctive nursing skills to take any notice of what was written on my medical notes in regard to the psychological analyses that I had been humiliatingly made to undergo when reporting the gynaecological symptoms. 'If she has psychological assessment on her notes, then what is her mental health diagnosis?', I overheard them discussing me.

'She doesn't have one. It just says that she has psychosomatic gynaecological symptoms due to possible depression.'

'Hmm. A psychiatrist commenting on gynae symptoms, and now she's being treated for cervical cancer? What a coincidence—not!'

The lead surgeon discussed the medical notes about the huge leakage during the night. She was concerned about the leakage and took me to an examination room at the far end of the corridor. Ethan, Meena, and the surgeon all carried the tubing, drips, and catheter bag as I walked slowly down the room and corridor. I couldn't feel where I was stepping properly but didn't want to complain about it. Ethan smiled as he said, 'You're doing brilliantly Beck! I can't believe you're up and about like this so soon!'. The surgeon seemed pleased in this respect too.

But she was clearly concerned with what was going on with the leakage and was very thorough in getting to the cause of it.

Ethan waited outside the examination room as the surgeon examined me, Meena assisting her. The fluid spilled out as I lay down, covering the examination couch and forming pools on the floor below.

The surgeon checked all of my abdominal and pelvic area, before concluding, 'Rebecka, the leakage is not from the bladder at all. This is lymphatic fluid; the largest loss I have seen.'

She went on to explain that the leakage of lymphatic fluid is called lymphorrhagia, and that it was coming from tiny openings called surgical channels to allow the fluid to flow around the body, rather than build up to dangerous levels following the removal of the lymph nodes. It was expected to slow down and cease altogether eventually, but for the next few weeks, it would continue to be a major issue.

The vast amount of lymphatic fluid that I lost added to my being even more unwell.

Whilst lymphatic impairment had been mentioned to me as a potential side effect of my cancer treatment, I had given it no more thought, thinking that as I was very fit, it would not affect me—and, while I was immensely grateful that I was actually not incontinent after all, it sunk in that we were actually dealing with something equally, or even more, distressing.

The surgeon told me that whilst this kind of reaction in the lymphatic system was rare, it was known to occasionally occur. The surgeon then left instructions with Meena as they discussed my care. Ethan spoke with the surgeon whilst Meena called an additional nurse in to help.

'She has had a *serious* lymph fluid loss,' said Meena to the other nurse. The nurse looked shocked as she stared at the huge pools of fluid covering the bed and floor.

'I've never seen anything like that before,' said the nurse, with a look of complete disbelief.

It had always been uncomfortable for me to be the exception to things so often and this was yet again just another aspect that was making me unusual.

I still could not get any rest. The cleaners were friendly and would speak nicely to me as they cleaned around my bedspace, but some other members of staff (not the doctors) would often gather by the entrance, which happened to be by my bedspace, during the only part of the day when there was supposed to be a short time of quietness. Their relentless loud chatter, combined with all the other constant noise, shouting, and sometimes threatening behaviour, was sensory overload, when all my body yearned to do was sleep-off the effects of the massive surgery.

Evening came with its visiting hours, which were supposed to be for three hours, but in reality, began at around two in the afternoon and prevailed all evening, until around eleven. The noise sounded similar to that of the crowd at a sports event, or what I imagined a disordered psychiatric institution to sound like—and did, according to Ethan, who had some experience of working in them.

It was late at night, and the visitors still hung around. The pandemonium and inquisitive, near-constant staring would only continue. A man who had been watching me looked around to see if anyone would notice and then made his way over to my bedspace. This time, I was more alert and able to shout out, 'No, *get away* from me,' A nurse told me off for my fleeting moment of expressing my distress, though it was uncharacteristic for me to ever do so and was done entirely in self-defence.

The visitors all left eventually, and the curtains were pulled around the beds at around midnight. At some point, completely exhausted, in the early hours I felt safe enough to fall asleep.

Early in the morning, I was awoken by the clattering of the curtain hooks being sharply pulled back.

'Come on. *Up,*' a nurse, who was pulling the curtains from around my bed, instructed.

I tried to stir.

'I'm not having you lying in bed all day; you can do things for yourself. You're a young, fit girl. When did you last get out of bed?'

'Last night,' I softly answered.

'You should be up and walking around everywhere.'

'But I do get up regularly,' I quietly pleaded, 'I'm sorry that I just can't manage to do that constantly; I am in such pain, and I can't feel the floor properly.'

As a self-disciplined, always motivated, always very active, and independent person for all of my life, I had tried all that I could to walk at regular intervals, but with the combination of the lymphatic problems and not having much feeling in my feet, the pain, and the morphine and catheter that I was attached to, along with the place being almost constantly full of loud, staring visitors, with their degrading commentary on me as I walked past them in my nightdress, this was challenging at the time for me.

'Look, you need to get up. I'm going to tell your surgeon that you refuse to walk or get up, and she will be very cross with you!

'But I don't refuse to walk,' I quietly begged in confusion. 'I have been out of bed and walking regularly since the surgery. I want to walk and to be able to do everything for myself again, but it's extremely difficult to do that all of the time. I am sorry that I can't.'

Suddenly, she threw back the bed covers. 'Get up', she said sharply, as she took hold of my feet and pulled me diagonally half out of bed. I let out a yelp of pain, which seemed to only make her more cross as she firmly responded, 'You silly girl! Getting upset *again*! We will refer you back to psychiatry for depression if you carry on.'

I do not think that she meant to hurt me in any way but was rather perhaps greatly ignorant to my full situation.

The pain seared through me, as I lay hanging out of the bed, feeling intense shame and humiliation. P*lease no,* I thought, *not again. Not those people that I had gotten away from with their repeated unnecessary analyses.* I wished that she knew that in fact, the only reason that I had ever had assessment with a psychiatrist in the first place was solely due to my not being believed about the pain and bleeding symptoms and that I had not received psychiatric treatment and no mental illness was found, but it was very clear that she would never have listened to me anyway even if I had been given the chance to explain.

I got through the day in some kind of numbed state of shock.

The evening passed in its usual pattern of my not only dealing with my pain and the leaking of my lymph fluid, but also with the usual shouting, disruptive and threatening behaviour and staring strangers standing around my bedspace. It was almost robotic; being shouted at and gawped at, or there for some to get the chance to speak to, according to what they were openly frequently discussing, an apparently appealing young woman, out of curiosity. The intolerable noise level overwhelmed my senses.

When Ethan came to see me, he looked ill himself: little to my knowledge at that time, he was enduring some horrid experiences of his own. It was one of the harshest British winters on record, and it came swift and unrelenting in its sub-zero bitterness. The building in which Ethan was staying, sleeping on the floor, was depressing, and outside of it, there was much drug use and crime. He had to constantly avoid being mugged, and he was cold and alone. He made sure to keep his plight largely concealed from me, but it was clear to see that he was suffering badly, and I felt intensely worried about him. For the first time since we had been together, there was nothing at all that I could do to help him.

Later that night, after he left, the usual visitors hung around and the mayhem continued for a while until most left and things were calming down—that is, until shouting and crashing noises came from further down the long room. It sounded like a man, a young one, was threatening people. *If a dangerous, violent situation is happening,* I thought, *I am stuck here; I can't get out. I can hardly move.*

At this commotion, a nurse came to mine and some other patients' bedsides with a worried expression. 'Don't be alarmed: it's a visitor. The police are on their way to remove him,' she explained. Apparently, he had become violent when realising he was expected to leave at the end of visiting hours. Nobody knew whether or not he was armed.

I sat anxiously in the hospital bed, hoping that he would not approach me. I knew that I would have to try and defend myself if he did, but then I realised that would be impossible in my condition.

A few minutes later, I sat in fear as police officers arrived and escorted the raging lad, who kicked anything in his path, past my bed and out of the building.

The shouting and aggression that occurred many times a day, along with the very chatoic environment, made me feel as though I would lose my mind. I just wanted it to stop. *Please, make it stop. Please.*

At some point the following morning, Ethan and the lead surgeon were stood over my bed, the surgeon wanting to do some speedy bloodwork, as she saw signs that my body was struggling to recover. She returned later to check on me and to look at my records for the latest blood test results and in doing so, told me, aghast and with deep concern, that among other things, the bloodwork had showed that my body was starving. The surgeon asked one of the nurses to fetch me a yoghurt from the catering staff, instructing Ethan to ensure that I ate it at once. She made sure that I had access to some food from then on—I could manage to eat only a little given that I was recovering from such extensive surgery—and then the nice tea lady began to bring me a hot chocolate in the evenings, both of these helping to build my strength a little.

Communicating my suffering to the doctors, who had all treated both myself and Ethan conscientiously and were not only brilliant in their work but also seemed to be lovely people, felt extremely difficult. Some were surgeons with very hectic working schedules, so I felt I could not burden them with my problems. Instead, I tried to address them smilingly and thank them for caring for me, being mindful of the pressures that they worked under. But secretly, I longed for them to notice how bad things were for me. Often whenever the doctors made their visits, however, the nurses made sure there were no visitors and everything was run as it should be for the time that the doctors were present, then things would change back to the usual conditions as soon as they left.

Later that day, I learned that a nurse, who would now not be at work for several days, had left recommendations that a physiotherapist come to me and help improve my walking. But this angered one of the other nurses, who glared at me with disdain, saying: 'It's *not* the physio's job to help you walk; you can do it yourself.' So, I tried to implement the training of the different disciplines that I had studied, to try to get myself back on my feet properly.

But I still could not fully feel the ground when I walked and had some numbness in my feet. Though I was getting out of bed and walking regularly, it felt strange adapting to my changed body in doing so. The angry nurses, however, refused to believe that I had any problem in this regard. To the contrary of their view, my lifelong unwavering self-discipline and determination not to give up had meant that (according to my surgeons) I was in fact doing a great deal to help myself to be up and about—much earlier than expected—and could not have been doing this any better.

It would later transpire that the reasons for the loss of some of the feeling in my feet, which at the time affected my walking, were most genuine and serious indeed. Some of the nurses did not properly understand or were even particularly aware of lymphoedema. Neither had they considered that I had what turned out to be nerve damage from the treatment for the cancer.

Even now, perhaps because I always looked like a very fit and healthy young woman—and one who was quiet and never made a fuss about anything—I was still not being listened to where my health was concerned. It was fine however: I was capable of looking after myself, but at times like these, it was tough to get by, having to adapt to such strange and new circumstances. Then again, the resilience that I had possessed since adolescence was my saviour right now: I mentally coached myself to adapt as much as possible without assistance.

The lymph leakage continued, and I was monitored for it now by my surgeons.

The loud disruption, shouting, and gawping from the visitors also continued as the days went by. The complete lack of privacy had marked me significantly: the violation of knowing that my body had been seen by strangers in such a way without my permission felt shatteringly degrading.

One evening, the bed opposite to mine became occupied by a very loud young woman and during her night there, she disrupted the place further. I knew what she was here for—I think the whole world did—as she was openly reciting on her mobile phone her apparently near-death experience: a very minor issue that had required a treatment lasting only a few minutes and she had no illness (as a doctor could be heard explaining to her). But you could tell that to her delight, she was going to get much mileage out of this for a long time to come. Her excitable blaring phone conversations, seemingly to everyone she had ever met, had been going on all evening and now into the middle of the night. For some reason, the nurses allowed her disruptive behaviour as she rang the nurses' alarm repeatedly for their attention, with them indulging her every whim and relentless vapid chatter. When she caught me looking in her direction in my pained state, she shouted, 'what?! I am really ill! I could have died!'.

This additional din was insufferable and in a futile attempt to try and drown some of it out, I covered my ears with my hands. But that is not really effective, and you can only do it for so long, so I went into the bathroom for some of the night; the only way, though not safe in my condition and a deeply unpleasant environment to be in, that I could escape the crazy behaviour and noise.

In the morning, the matriarch of the nice family came over to chat to me. She told me that she was concerned by how I was treated and by my being mostly alone. I found it difficult to talk to her, given how affected I was by the situation that I was in, but I appreciated that a stranger expressed genuine empathy towards me. She came back to say goodbye to me when her daughter left later that day.

When I was next visited by the surgeon, I begged her to let me leave. At first, she said that my lymph fluid loss and blood pressure readings had to return to more normal levels before she could do that. Upon my pleading with her again the next day, the surgeon, who trusted Ethan's experience as a medic, agreed to let me go home with the assistance of her precise care instructions being thoroughly implemented.

On the final evening that I spent at that place with its crazy, unruly atmosphere, I willed myself through the usual unbearably loud noise levels, staring faces, and lecherous or threatening attempts to approach me from some of the visitors, trying to focus my mind on the knowledge that I would very soon be getting out of there.

In the morning, it was arranged for me to be discharged to go home. Ethan called the person who was assigned to oversee my care to check on what time the medical vehicle for my return journey would arrive, as this had been agreed to beforehand, and she was aware that I had no way of getting back otherwise. A nurse came to me and said, 'A medical vehicle will be ready for you in half an hour, but your partner isn't allowed in it. If he has to let you in the house, then tell him to go home now, or he won't be back in time, and you'll be left waiting outside.'

To be left outside alone in my condition in the freezing weather could put me in life-threatening circumstances, so on her advice, I phoned Ethan from the nursing station and repeated what the nurse had told me. He thought I would be looked after, so gathered himself in a rush, dashing out of the building and to the train station to get home in time to let me in. He called me just as he boarded, immediately after which the nurse came back to ask me if my partner was on the train..

'Yes, he's on the train now,' I replied.

'Well,' she said with a smug look, 'he could have come with you after all.'

I was bewildered at why she would relish my now being fully alone in my helpless state. But I continued to be utterly respectful towards her and the other nurses as I felt that I always had to be polite.

Another came to me, looking nervous. 'The ambulance vehicle that you were meant to have was not arranged for you properly,' she said apologetically. 'So, you can't get home that way.'

The news that I was stuck there, surrounded by danger, totally alone and unable to get home, was daunting. I tried to figure out what to do in my frightening, solitary, completely vulnerable predicament,

Fiona joined me between her tasks, seeming concerned. 'I'm sorry that you have no way of getting home. The person overseeing your care should be arranging something for you with another medical vehicle, but we can't get through to her'.

Gina brought all the medication that I would need to take home with me, including the morphine and the anticoagulant injections being administered into my abdomen, the catheter tubing and bags, dressings, and all the other necessary medical paraphernalia. There was so much stuff that I seemed to be surrounded by bags of kit by the time we were done. Gina removed the cannula, which having been the largest size of IV needle due to the scale of the surgery, seemed huge on my slim wrist. It left a wound, that would forever remain as a small scar, which she covered with a dressing. Then, she strapped the catheter bag to my thigh.

Hours went by as I sat alone, and the medical vehicle still had not arrived. A pleasant nurse who I had not seen before came to me but had to leave quickly for her duties. 'Hello, lovely! I was here on the day of your surgery, and I have been on holiday since. You won't remember me, but I looked after you when you came back from theatre. You've done really well getting through all that so soon.' Despite the nurses who had treated me with utter contempt, a few others had been most conscientious in their care and had been kind when speaking to me.

It was now time for Gina to leave, and she sat beside me, looking very concerned. 'Rebecka, please call us when you get back. I'm worried about you. I'm leaving now, but I will want to know how you are and if you get back safely.' As she rose to leave, she embraced me, which took me by surprise. She seemed to know some of what I had been going through but looked helpless to do anything about it. I comprehended her situation and the stress being placed on her in her job and felt sympathetic towards her circumstances.

The usual men continued pretending to wash their hands by the bed, staring at me as they did so. Now that I was alert and felt some hope at the prospect of leaving, I told them sternly, through my distress, to leave me alone whenever they attempted to approach me. However, this appeared to have the opposite effect: hearing my different voice just seemed to pique their interest even more.

Day turned to early evening, and a man wandered into the room, calling, 'Taxi? Taxi?'

I heard the angry nurse say, 'That's for her.'

She looked at me and snapped, 'Go on, then! Go!'

A mixture of confusion and apprehension filled me, as I softly tried to explain to her, 'But the medical car...'

'You're not having a medical car,' the nurse snapped. 'You don't need one. There's hardly anything wrong with you, silly girl'

I looked at the tubes, catheter bag, and medical paraphernalia attached to me, as well as the heavy bags of medical kit, knowing that I was going to have to suddenly manage all of this completely alone. I was on morphine and, although I could now walk slowly and unaided for a very short distance, I was still incapacitated and the full feeling in my feet had not returned. I was also classed as in a thirty-day 'danger period' of risk of life-threatening side effects due to the extent of the surgery that I had received, and the surgeon had emphasised how seriously that needed to be addressed. These challenges felt most daunting indeed, in this place of being surrounded by an undercurrent of menace.

Faced with the sudden situation of having to leave alone in a taxi, that had no medical support for my serious immediate medical needs, outside among the threatening behaviour and then in a journey across a motorway in treacherous winter weather, I became frightened. But the nurse was completely unsympathetic.

My instinct was always absolutely to flee the place, but in this situation, I knew logically that it would be even more dangerous for me outside, where people were sometimes openly mugged in broad daylight and in front of everyone, than it was here.

'Please, I don't know how I will manage in this condition. I can't move about properly', I quietly pleaded.

'Not my problem. You're discharged; you're off my hands now', she said.

I of course desperately wanted to leave the place, but, the fact was that in my condition, I needed help to do so and as well as it being dangerous for me to be making my way out of there alone in my completely vulnerable state, the entrance to the building was some distance away considering my condition (in normal circumstances, it would be absolutely no problem to walk there whatsoever), it would be impossible for me to walk that distance in my state of health, having received such major surgery.

'I can't get to the entrance,' I softly and politely tried to explain. 'I am struggling to walk. I don't know what I am going to do.'

'Like I said, not my problem', she answered scornfully. 'I don't know what you want me to do about it.' *Go on'*, she sternly ordered, as she waived her hand towards the door.

Though I was frightened at my immediate quite alarming situation, knowing that I had to try and safely get through it sharply focused the mind, so I did the best that I could to adapt to it.

I struggled to lift all the bags of medical kit. The taxi driver took some, however.

I looked at the floor, trying to feel where I was stepping as I silently walked toward the doorway of the room. I slowly made my way down the long corridor that entered the floors leading to the ground floor, the reception area, then the entrance and then to the carpark. The taxi driver, though he was nice enough, went on ahead and kept shouting over from further down the corridor for me to hurry up as he was in a rush being on a time schedule. The lymph fluid leakage continued as I walked and began seeping through my clothing. Pain seared through me, and I struggled to walk this far, especially when I could not fully feel where I was stepping and with the tubing attached to me. *Come on, you can get through it, deal with the pain with each step,* I coached myself mentally.

Those visitors who had been preying on the combination of my girlish femininity and intense vulnerability, now began to seize their chance to try and touch me. One grinned as he tried to talk to me and get close, a couple of others were looking around to assess the situation. I felt frightened and tremblingly realised that they might be about to actually get hold of me. I walked further than I had since the surgery and felt more agonising pain with each and every step. The next thing I knew, I lost my balance, and I was lying on the floor in the corridor, in even more pain.

Almost immediately, a nurse who I had never seen before was suddenly rushing around me, trying to help. 'Are you okay?' I heard her ask. I tried to answer through the pain and mumbled something. She looked at my wristband, which had my name on it. 'Are you okay, Rebecka?'.

The nurse asked what department I had come from. 'Have you had surgery?' she asked, noticing the tubing attached. 'What are you doing out here on your own?' I briefly mentioned radical surgery, for treatment of cancer, wincing with pain as I spoke.

She looked dismayed and held my hand as I lay on the floor. She introduced herself as Chloe. She checked the catheter and whether I was bleeding from my wounds. Intense embarrassment over my predicament, along with the pain, overcame me.

As she spoke to a passing nurse from the department where I had come from, it transpired that Chloe worked in an adjacent part of the building. The nurse that she spoke to about me had not mistreated me in any way and had been conscientious of my care when she had been looking after me but perhaps had not been fully aware of what was happening to me. I could not quite hear most of the conversation between them, but it was apparent that Chloe was expressing her disgust at my having been discharged in my condition alone, without any assistance and that, according to her, I showed signs of neglect. It was decided that Chloe would look after me from then on, as she was informed that I could not be taken anywhere else in the building—and, with that, she fetched a wheelchair and helped me into it.

We went into the lift to the ground floor and then through the corridors, with Chloe checking on me all the while. I looked at the floor as she gently tried to get me to open up about what I had been going through. I had a terrible fear that I would not be believed if I dared mention what I had experienced, but Chloe told me that the fact that she had found me alone in a corridor in such an unprotected and fragile state said it all. She seemed to fully understand what had been happening to me and spoke to me in a gentle manner but was clearly perturbed and angry by what she had observed, urging me to report it.

'I'm disgusted,' she fretted. 'I don't want to have to go along with this and put you alone in a taxi to travel across the motorway in your condition, especially in this weather, but I've been left with no choice.' She was especially concerned upon learning that I did not have a mobile phone, and so nobody would be aware if, on the journey back home, I got into danger or took a turn for the worse with the side effects from the surgery.

She pushed me in the hospital wheelchair to the entrance of the building and outside, where the taxi was. The cold outside was biting in its harshness, with snow coating the ground and a blizzard beginning. Chloe was wearing a short-sleeved tunic and must have felt the cold badly, but she took the time to place me into the old and uncomfortable vehicle, doing so carefully, before taking one last check of all the tubes and medical equipment. She had an expression of great concern.

Before she closed the door, she clutched my hand with purpose and with most seriousness said, 'You promise me that you will report what has happened to you. You can do it confidentially. If you don't, nothing will ever get changed. Please promise me,' she pleaded.

'I don't want to, but I promise you that I will,' I responded. 'Thank you so much for helping me. I don't know what I would have done without your help. I'm so grateful to you.'

She gently squeezed my hand with affection, 'tell your partner to call us when you get back so that we know you have arrived safely. *Please* make sure that he does, Rebecka, or I will worry.'

And with that, Chloe and I waved at one another as the car pulled away, my hands trembling with nervousness.

Although it would happen that I would never have the opportunity to see or speak to Chloe again, I would never forget how she had come to my aid that day, and how incredibly conscientious she was in her role as a nurse (I have thought about her since and hope that she is having a nice life).

Now, I had a new fear to contend with: the long journey home, alone apart from the stranger who was the taxi driver, having to manage my immediate severe medical needs and pain, through the outside threatening behaviours and along the ice-covered motorway during a freezing blizzard, in the dark. It was strange and unnerving being in this state—that is, one almost as vulnerable as a human being can be.

As we drove past menacing gangs of people hanging around, I

was afraid: I was completely at the mercy of anyone who felt like taking advantage of my incapacitated state.

As we approached the motorway, queues of traffic were being managed by the police due to the dangerous weather conditions and there were hazard lights flashing. The snow had formed a heavy blizzard, and the roads were icy. The car that I was in was not modern and quite cold and very uncomfortable with hard seats that put pressure on the swollen and post-surgical parts of my body, increasing the level of pain that I was in.

Later that evening, Ethan was stunned to find the taxi driver knocking on the front door of our house, as he had no knowledge of what had occurred, believing that a medical vehicle was bringing me home, as he had been assured by the nursing support person. He came out to the taxi, helping me out carefully.

'I'm shocked that they let you go out there on your own in all of that danger and have sent you home in a taxi by yourself. It's icy everywhere; how do they expect me to get you into the house in your condition?', he said. But we managed, though I nearly fell a couple of times, with very careful tiny steps along the road and down the path. We eventually made it back inside the house.

Now back at home, the degradation that I felt was intense, though I could not express it, only tremblingly breaking down a little.

Though distressed, in much pain, and completely emotionally shattered, I lay silently in my bed with a feeling of overwhelming relief as I took in the realisation that I had survived—and not only that, but that I had made it back against all the odds, in every sense.

11

But I Did Try to Tell You...

THE FOLLOWING TWO WEEKS WERE spent recovering at home, and as the unusually harsh sub-zero winter weather continued, I was then taken by ambulance in the icy conditions to be admitted for further medical care at the local hospital for the effects of the cancer.

At this point, I had no idea how affected I was by what I had cumulatively been through. I would frequently wake up in the night with a start, thinking I was locked in a building, immobile, and at the mercy of any unscrupulous person. While during the day, particular noises would startle me. For several weeks after the surgery, I was given a daily injection into my abdominal area, to manage the risk of immediate heart problems and blood clotting due to the severity of the surgery. During one of these, I suddenly had a flash back when the nurses leaned over me to administer the injection and became quite upset. Some of the nurses picked up on my traumatised state and spoke to me about it but I would not tell them much at all: at this time, I found it difficult to speak to people and was quite withdrawn.

The nurses immediately nicknamed me 'Tinkerbell', since they felt that I was 'fairy-tale' looking. I was still to apparently be 'Sleeping Beauty' to those on the other small ward that I was sometimes in for surgical care, but here, I was 'Tinkerbell'. As I certainly did not think that I was like a fairy-tale character, I simply found these monikers to be humorous, as they were meant affectionately. But it was ironic that I had been viewed in this way when my life could not have been any less fairytale-like.

While in hospital, the catheter was removed to allow me to undergo a trial without it under observation. It felt wonderful to be free of the bag and tubing.

A few hours later, I felt an acute pain in my lower back and pelvic area. I told a nurse about this, and she explained that it was the result of the bladder attempting to work again on its own. The nurse helped me to walk to the bathroom, and then I suddenly felt myself slump forward.

The pain was excruciating, and I doubled over, crying out in agony. It took something utterly dreadful and life threatening for me ever to make any kind of fuss. Other nurses rushed to me. One of the medical team shouted, 'Get a catheter into her *now*.'

I could process nothing but this unbelievable pain as I writhed around in agony.

The nurses were swift in dealing with what had almost become an emergency situation requiring surgery and attached the catheter immediately. I felt an instantaneous relief from the pain, and my noise calmed. I lay motionless and exhausted but could now take in the bleeping machinery around me.

'Are you alright there, Tinkerbell?' asked a nurse. 'That was a close one! Your body didn't like that at all. We've replaced the catheter now, so you should start to feel better.'

As the agonising pain quickly subsided, I began to feel embarrassed at all the commotion I had caused.

Being back in a medical establishment so soon had evoked raw memories in me, and I particularly struggled at night, when I had nightmares and felt nervous constantly. Sudden noises would often startle me, in my new near-constant state of hypervigilance.

After a few days of my stay, the nurses grew concerned when seeing me alone at visiting times when Ethan could not be there as he had to work, though he would visit when he wasn't working, He worked very long hours in a poorly paid and unpleasant job that was detrimental to his health and which he yearned to leave—having been repeatedly denied the opportunity to work in his civilian profession due to a lack of access to training and support— sometimes getting little sleep in the process and cycling there and back in all weathers. He carried on the best he could and completely independently, despite his own problems that he had faced since leaving the military. But I felt very sad for his situation and hoped that I could be of help to him in improving it in the future and I wanted so much better for him.

But not seeing anyone, apart from Ethan, was really okay. I was fine on my own because knowing that those where I came from would revel in my circumstances if discovering how dreadful they were—though I was used to that and could handle it emotionally—I did not want to have to deal with or listen to that particular behaviour at this incredibly challenging time of my life. All in all, being alone, even at this turbulent and agonising time of my life when I had been so ill and faced the possibility of losing my life and was in dire circumstances, was infinitely better than having to put up with some others' ridicule, gloating and glee at seeing me end up just as they had always ordered me to be; in their view, hiding any qualities that I might have, not being seen or heard, a nothingness.

Most people have a network of others around them for support for much of or the entirety of their lives. I had never had that. But not only had I never felt the need for that (as they say, what you never have, you never miss), I also always felt that I was not the only person in the world to be in such a position in regard to this particular aspect.

Apart from that side of things however, it was bad luck that I had very briefly met lovely people in the arts who were kind and friendly towards me and we enjoyed being in each other's company, but my circumstances meant that I was very rarely able to be around them (and I could not just tell people that I did not know well what was happening to me as that would be too bizarre and dramatic to convey). Therefore, I never got to know anyone properly.

Some good news arrived: a nurse came to see me to tell me that the results of the lymph node dissection element of my surgery had been received. 'They're clear, Rebecka,' she said, looking immensely happy, as she held my hand affectionately.

I felt ecstatic with relief to learn that the metastasis had been stopped in its tracks and that the cancer had most likely been prevented from spreading any further. I had been previously informed that this optimal scenario with the cancer was highly unlikely, as the tumour had begun to spread towards the local lymphatic nodes and bladder—but, as we would now realise, miraculously, my body had, for twelve years, managed to sort of keep in check the tumour, which, so I was told, had been caught just in the nick of time, before it entered the lymph nodes.

The intuitive female doctor who had, at that chance appointment, intervened with the issues with my medical care to investigate the symptoms further and discovered my cancer, essentially saved my life, something that was later confirmed by some medics.

My two surgeons were also responsible for my still being here, of course. One of them phoned the hospital ward and wanted to speak to me personally to tell me about the news and explain everything to me. She told me that while they were confident that they had removed all of the cancer, I would never be given the all-clear because of its high-grade nature; rather, I would simply (hopefully) always remain in remission. Serious complications aside, however, where the cancer was concerned, it had been the best outcome we could have hoped for, and the specialists felt that they had treated it as successfully as possible.

I told my surgeon how I could not have wished for a better theatre team. 'I really mean this: thank you from the bottom of my heart for saving my life.'

'That's okay, darling,' she answered affectionately. 'That's what we're here for. We don't do it for the money; it's the ability to help save lives that motivates us. There's no better feeling to us in what we do than providing a good outcome, and the research in your case will help us to provide more of them.'

I was touched that she had taken the time out of her busy day to personally call me and have a chat; how fortunate I was to have been treated by two of the most highly-skilled surgeons for my particular oncological case.

Knowing that my unusual circumstances, which I had often felt uncomfortable about, had at least benefitted cancer research in such a way, was some comfort to me.

The news of my remission from cancer did not involve

celebration or the ringing of a bell or anything like that; I had to quietly get on with my life and began to deal with the consequences of what I had survived and the very tough circumstances that I found myself in.

After leaving hospital again, I spent a few weeks at home, but being there now presented other challenges: the house, though always clean and tidy, had grown to be neglected in terms of repairs over the last few years as a result of our lack of income due to my illness, and its old, thin windows were deteriorating and in the freezing conditions of such a harsh winter, they were icing over on the inside. We had never had the chance financially to improve the very old bathroom, either, which had only a bath and no shower, and was permanently icy cold in the winter. Now, in my newly heavily post-surgical and painful state, with a very long recovery ahead of me, these circumstances at home were extremely uncomfortable to manage with—but I struggled on.

Due to return to the local hospital for further care of the catheter and post-surgical issues, an ambulance was scheduled to collect me that morning but did not show up. Hours later, there was still no sign of the ambulance and now Ethan was forced to leave for work, otherwise being at risk of losing his job. But he had been assured by the hospital that the ambulance would be there imminently, so we both expected that I would not be alone for more than around twenty minutes at the most. Therefore, it did not seem like I was in any danger when he had to leave.

Alone at home, I sat, waiting for the ambulance to arrive as the hours went by. I was due a dosage of morphine. I began to feel severe pain—not just from the area of the surgery and my swollen abdomen, but in the area of my kidneys. This pain gradually worsened, and I tentatively stood from the sofa to move to a more comfortable position but fell to the floor. I let out a shriek of pain.

There were problems with the catheter that needed to be dealt with urgently.

The pain was becoming agonising.

Darkness was descending outside as the winter's early evening crept in. I was lying on the floor, in pain, with no lights on in the house.

Then, I heard voices not too far away: people walking down the front garden path. This was then followed by a knock at the door.

'Hello!' I tried to shout back, as agonising pain seared through me. They knocked again. 'Hello! Help!' I shouted louder.

The front door was old and thin, so the ambulance medics were able to hear me through it. 'Rebecka are you there?' they called.

'Yes, I'm here! I'm going to try and get to the door,' I answered, wincing with pain.

I could see that the medics were peering through the window, and one of them went to get a torch to see in the dark. The light of the torch shone through the window onto me.

I dragged myself across the floor on my hands and knees, whimpering with pain as I did so. It took all of my strength to very slowly get onto my feet, holding onto the wall, reach up, and somehow, in stages, open the heavy lock on the door.

When I did, I cried out in agony. The ambulance medics came rushing in, dealing with the situation immediately and took me back to the local hospital.

It was just another in a long list of degrading experiences that I wondered were ever going to end.

Once again attempting to remove the medical equipment attached to my bladder, I was referred for a consultation with a urological surgeon.

My recovery continued between home and the local hospital over the next few months as the New Year came and went, I continued to endure the uncomfortable conditions at home and particularly struggled with the freezing old bathroom and its lack of a shower, as I was recovering from the effects of the cancer treatment.

Though the lymphorrhagia continued, it had slowed right down in its flow. The feeling in my feet meanwhile still had not returned fully, and I struggled with this when I walked and was concerned that it was going to inhibit my recovery and regaining of my fitness.

One day, attempting at some exercises with my feet, determined that I would return to dance, I recalled what I had been told, in that I might never be able to be a dancer again due to the effects of the cancer treatment.

In my focus for survival, I had not fully considered the lasting consequences of the cancer treatment. Now, I was having to face them head-on, as I was living with them.

My instinctive feeling that something did not add up with the correlation between the discovery of my tumour and my symptoms of pain and bleeding nagged away at me, and I ruminated over it during my days at home. Clearly now, something had not been right; something had gone very wrong.

Following this conclusion, I was advised to speak with a legal representative to express my concerns. I had no hard evidence at this stage—just a hunch and a timeline of events that seemed to suggest that I may have had the tumour for a long time.

Just three months after the radical surgery, I was found to have complications and underwent further surgery to help correct them. My body felt so tender from all of the treatment, and it was painful.

Whilst in hospital, I managed to take a better look at my medical notes, being that they were by my bed, and was stunned at what I read: the psychiatrist's opinion, though without an actual diagnosis, had counted for everything, and was still continuing to influence my medical care; practically everything that I said and did in a medical professionals' presence was recorded in my notes and psycho-analysed due to this.

I was devastated to discover that this had been determined entirely on the basis of my cervical screening tests being clear and that when no clinical explanation could be found for my symptoms, a psychiatrist had been sent to see me to try and establish if they were therefore psychological. He had searched into my childhood to find a reason why I may be apparently 'imagining' the symptoms—and, upon learning that I had been a poor and abused adolescent, he had almost cast me off effectively as a product of my unfortunate early years, despite there never being any issues with my mind or development.

(Much later, when I would further be able to read through my medical notes as part of the legal proceedings, it would be hurtful to discover that among the very complementary way that some of the doctors had kindly described me as a person, there were other comments from a few medical professionals, some of whom I had trusted in revealing a little of what had happened to me in my medical care, that openly mocked my reporting of the misdiagnosis).

After I had undergone my latest surgery, the original gynaecologist-oncologist came to see me in the hospital, accompanied by two nurses. He discussed my treatment and the effects of it, and I took this as an opportunity to try and explain how badly affected I was by what I had been through with the effects of the misdiagnosis. But he simply said, 'Just try to forget about it. You can just go back to being normal now' and then, referencing the psychoanalysis that I had been wrongly referred for following my reporting of the pain and bleeding symptoms and my (only very briefly mentioned upon questioning) deprived and abusive early years, added dryly, 'or as normal as you ever were'. Previously, the consultant had been very complimentary about my demeanour and conduct, in person and in writing in medical correspondence to other doctors and in my medical notes. But now, having learned the full extent of the unfortunate circumstances I had faced, of which had been beyond my control, including throughout the misdiagnosis, his opinion of me had changed to become seemingly one of ridicule. This humiliating reaction only added to the implication that too much of an unwarranted interest had been taken in me from a psychoanalytical point of view, especially given the fascination with psychiatry by certain doctors.

A few weeks after this, I saw the same consultant for a check-up, only for my complications to be left unacknowledged as he deemed these issues to be 'non-specific'.

I tried to broach with him that which I had read in my medical notes, asking him if the pain and bleeding symptoms that I had suffered from for many years could have had anything to do with the tumour, but he quickly dismissed my concerns. However, he told me that a review of my tests was being done by an independent organisation as a matter of procedure.

Hence, from this point, all I could do was continue my slow recuperation as winter turned into spring—and what a glorious spring it was, completely in contrast to the bitterly harsh winter we had just experienced: the sun shone brightly, and the warmth provided me with great relief from the cold in the house. Ethan still had to work most of the time, and so, at the time, still being unable to walk properly, I was not able to go out of the house much. We did not have a proper garden to sit in, either. But I relished every moment of being in nature and seeing flowers come into bloom, and, having that feeling of being involved in life again, as I began to take short walks on my own.

Later in the summer, Ethan and I were shopping in a mall. I had never been keen on shopping centres but now found that I had developed a discomfort in this type of environment. As we were walking around, I became more and more uncomfortable, as though my senses were overwhelmed, and felt stressed in a way which was completely out of character for me. But I could not explain why I suddenly felt that way: the lights; the noise; the lights; the noise; people chattering and shouting... I ended up trying to flee the building, but, of course, in my condition at the time, did not get very far.

At first, Ethan could not understand what was wrong with me, as I had never behaved like this before. With his life experience, it did not take long for him to figure out what was going on. 'You know how you were denied trauma therapy after the surgery?' he approached one day. 'I think it might be good for you to talk about that with your doctor; I think you are traumatised by what has happened to you over the last few years.'

Brushing this off, I told him that I was fine; that I could handle it. But he persisted that I should at least mention it to my new, very understanding doctor.

Placing even more effort into retraining my body and trying to exercise, I found that it was a painfully slow process. In light of this struggle, I was sent to physiotherapy —but I still did not regain full feeling in my feet. They felt that I may have sustained some nerve damage during the treatment for the cancer. However, I would not give up on keeping fit, and so, despite the pain I was in, I did whatever exercise I could manage nearly every day. I willed myself to keep persevering; carry on, moving my body in any way I could, however painful, in an attempt to keep the fit and toned physique that was all I had ever identified with.

Just over a year after the diagnosis of the cancer, I was asked to come to the hospital for a review meeting with the consultant. I still did not quite know what to make of the consultant, as I found that his behaviour could veer between strange and inappropriate in terms of his words, to humiliating comments, and then to fleeting displays of seeming compassion, along with his interest in psycho-analysis.

Ethan accompanied me to the review meeting. There was a nurse in the department also in attendance. The consultant explained that an independent review of my cervical screening tests had been carried out as a matter of procedure. This review, he said, had shown repeated errors.

He had a report before him, which he read out to me. It stated that the most recent test had shown that I had cancer—something I already knew, since that had been the result to diagnose me—whilst the test three years previously also showed established cancer. He then continued that the test three years before that had also been positive for cancer. Then, finally, he said that the test from years before that—my first test of this kind—had shown that cancer was forming.

I tried to take in the shock of what I was hearing, as I lowered my head in disbelief.

The consultant, once he had finished reading this information out, leaned right back on his chair and asked with a look of intense anticipation, as he chewed on the end of a pen 'How does that make you feel?' oddly almost excitedly awaiting my response.

I paused for what seemed like a long time, not knowing how to answer. 'Well, I don't know how I feel about this,' I finally replied. I really did not know how I felt or how to respond apart from feeling shocked and dismayed.

'What are you going to do about it?' he asked, looking intently curious, while chewing on the end of a pen.

'I don't know,' was all I could reply at that stunned moment.

But then, after a long pause, I felt a surge of emotion at the thought of the pain, humiliation and loss of being able to do anything profound with the best years of my life, due to the misdiagnosis for so many years and so I managed to find the words to sincerely say, 'If you will forgive my forthrightness in saying this... for more than twelve years, I was repeatedly told that I was imagining the symptoms of pain and bleeding. I was told that it was all in my mind. A psychiatrist was asked to establish if my pain and bleeding was psychological, given that the cervical screening test results were normal, and so he probed into my childhood as part of an assessment to find reasons why I might have supposed psychosomatic physical symptoms—and from this he then stated that I was interpreting unacknowledged emotional pain from childhood as physical pain, and so probably had depression. They would not believe me. Though they couldn't find any mental illness, they made me undergo completely unnecessary repeated psychoanalysis to keep trying to find something, anything, that they could pinpoint my reporting of the pain and bleeding to. They suggested that I could be forcibly given antidepressant treatment for no reason other than the pain and bleeding being deemed as psychosomatic due to possible depression. I lost any chance I ever had of building my work in the arts because of this; I had overcome my deprived start to build my way up to that and then had those opportunities taken away from me. I lost what should have been the best years of my life, and almost my life, entirely because some people believed that their opinions must be correct, or they misused their position all on the basis of a theory.'

As I finished speaking, I immediately regretted releasing such an outpouring of emotion; my words, flowing from a heavy heart, now seemed irrelevant somehow.

'So, you feel vilified, because you were right?' asked the consultant with intense interest.

'It is not a question of my being right,' I softly and politely answered, 'it is the fact that I was not believed for all of those years for absolutely no reason, all because it was discovered that I had an abusive and neglectful early life.'

I felt suddenly compelled to query something that had been troubling me, and so added in a respectful tone, 'If I may please say so: what about those responsible for the tests? One wrong test I could put down to human error and unquestioningly forgive, but *three*, with a misdiagnosis over twelve years. I do not understand how that is possible due to simple error.'

However, I tried to bear in mind that, to their credit, although the health services effectively allowed my cancer to develop and caused the consequent health problems that I now had to live with for the rest of my life, they were also efficient in treating it once it had been diagnosed by new medics, so I sincerely thanked the consultant for the treatment that I had been given.

Ethan had kept silent during the entirety of this conversation but was visibly perturbed at the new information. The consultant looked at him and held his hands up. 'It's nothing to do with me, the testing,' he said.

The nurse shot the consultant an open-mouthed stare at that statement. There is no suggestion that the consultant was involved in any wrongdoing. But though Ethan and I maintained our usual politeness, we knew that there was more to this than was being disclosed to us, particularly in terms of the highly irregular situation of the incompetent testing that I was involved in and with certain aspects of clinical practice; there was much about the whole situation that remained a mystery, especially as nobody would discuss particular crucial elements of it and from the very strange comments that the consultant had made to me.

The consultant continued with an attempt at further psychoanalytical questions relating to the cancer and misdiagnosis—but as far as I was concerned, there was nothing more to say: for well over a decade, I had pleaded for help for my symptoms of pain and bleeding, only to be told repeatedly that they were psychosomatic and it was only now, more than thirteen years after the symptoms had first appeared, that my suffering had been proven to be attributable to genuine physical illness: cancer.

How could this just be a simple mistake? All of those tests being wrong and all of those psychological assessments that I had never needed. I thought.

It was apparent that I was now deeply involved in something possibly strange and irregular.

12

In the Dark

I T IS SOMETIMES DIFFICULT TO know how to navigate a world where you often feel you cannot fit in simply as a result of the downright darkness and bizarreness of the experiences that circumstances have forced you to endure.

That darkness and bizarreness, however, was only to become worse.

But I truly believe that we can learn from the darkest of times. That is what developing ourselves in terms of character is all about, and that is always within our grasp.

The meeting with the consultant—particularly his reaction to the review of my cervical screening tests—confirmed my suspicions that something possibly disturbing and irregular had happened. This was not a conclusion that I arrived at lightly; all along, I had been keen to give the benefit of the doubt to all of those involved in the matter, and I could certainly forgive honest mistakes and simple human error. But now, as I gathered all the relevant information, it was obvious that this could not possibly have been down to a simple mistake; indeed, it became apparent that this was something significantly wrong that I was involved in. Feeling overwhelmed by the situation that I had been placed in, after much consideration over what I should do, I felt I had no choice but to seek some legal advice to assist me in unravelling what had been happening with my medical care, since nobody involved seemed willing to be open with me about it.

Upon receiving the outcome of the cervical screening review, a legal representative commented, 'That's *really* bad.'

Meanwhile, the other matter of the confidential reporting of the hideous experiences at the place of the life-changing surgery that I had been urged, by some of the good nurses, to do, had come to nothing in the form of a contemptuous response of a good telling-off for raising the matter (prior to this, I actually hadn't been sure what the point was in saying anything about it in any case) and a thinly-veiled warning that if I tried to take any legal action—something that I had not even thought about doing anyway, especially as I had enough to contend with in that respect with the misread testing and misdiagnosis—about what I had been subjected to, I would be squashed in this respect. Distraught by this, I now wished that I had never spoken to anyone about what had happened to me. I was separately advised that, despite the repeated violations of my dignity, attempts of assault and threatening behaviour from the visitors, being found on the floor in the corridor, having to make my own way home alone in a heavily post-surgical state in dangerous circumstances, and so forth, it would all merely be classified as 'a distressing incident' as a whole and that any further action would be seen as pointless because the experiences would apparently not be considered to have done me any lasting harm.

Hence, feeling afraid of what would happen if I took the matter further, as well as the intense embarrassment that I felt at having endured such bizarre and degrading experiences, along with having spent my entire life avoiding being involved in any kind of fuss, I accepted the fact that I had to get over it: such is life.

The research that I had been involved in, of which I had, though fearful and forgoing some of my privacy, agreed to allow my body to be used for as a rare case to improve female cancer care, I of course, still hoped helped to save other lives. However, this element of my experiences had become a feature of my nightmares, in addition to those 'trapped' ones that I also had and those of people shouting at me and not believing me regarding the cancer symptoms. These nightmares often involved parts of my body, in a clinical sense, being on film and in a scientific laboratory, with the addition of being surrounded by people loudly questioning me (the shouting people being symbolic, not, of course, of my wonderful surgical team and brilliant surgeons, but of those who had confronted me with aggression and questioning during my misdiagnosis and also since the treatment for the cancer) – being nightmares of course, such things are distorted from how we view them when we are in consciousness. I worried that these weird images, displayed starkly in snapshots in my dreams, were an indication that I had lost my mind. I later learned that, in fact, such depictions during sleep are part of how the mind processes a traumatic event and are therefore the normal course of things and not a sign of insanity.

By this point, the full feeling in my feet had not yet returned since the surgery and therefore I was finally referred to the physiotherapy department. By now, I could manage to walk alone again, but I still had difficulty feeling where I was stepping. On one occasion, alone at home and attempting to get downstairs, I could not feel the steps under my feet and consequently fell from the top to the bottom of the full flight of them. I lay in a heap of agonising pain at the foot of the stairs, having also sustained small injuries and bruising from the fall and which required medical treatment. I stayed there like that for a little while, at the foot of the stairs, the humiliation and frustration of my circumstances overcoming me and I felt ashamed to be shedding tears for myself.

It turned out that there was little that the physiotherapy department could do for me, ultimately, as scans revealed extensive internal scar tissue, and it also became apparent that there was swelling to my legs and abdomen, along with some nerve damage. These were side effects of the surgery that had treated the cancer and so all I could do was learn to adapt to the way my body now functioned.

I tried as much as I could to do this, and I continued to persevere with rebuilding an exercise regime, despite my finding it very painful. Being physically active was the only way of life and state of my body that I had ever known, and now here I was, in very unfamiliar territory, finding it painful to walk and without the full feeling in my feet. I constantly pressed on, however, determined that I would re-train my body and was not going to let the effects of the cancer treatment take over my life.

It was shortly after this that a strange medical letter arrived, the first of quite a few—and, when I opened and began to read it, my heart began to beat fast, and I had a feeling of complete dread. At first, I could not quite believe the letter's contents. It was from both the consultant and a psychiatrist. It was bizarre as a whole, requesting that I attend a department that I had never been to before for psychological assessment for the purposes of research, relating to the psychological effects of the cancer that I had survived.

This inept request was even more emphasised by the accompanying questions I was asked, since their contents were strange at best: one of the questions was how I thought I would react to being in a disaster situation. I was also asked again, 'how do you react to stress?'. Despite the fact that the cervical screening review had clearly proven that my pain and bleeding had been attributable to cancer, I was *still* being psycho-analysed for my reasons for reporting the symptoms, and now for my response to the cancer diagnosis itself. *Why are they doing this?* I wondered. *Why, being as it has been concluded and confirmed that I don't have mental illness, can't they just cease questioning me about the way I think, feel and react to things?* They just could not seem to understand how someone from my incredibly deprived and abused early years could have strength, resilience, any depth of character and not to have turned to addiction or bad behaviour, quite the opposite of what is taught in some traditional psychiatry, and their curiosity in this respect often suggested that they seemed somewhat creepily almost fascinated by how I had turned out to be so very different to that.

The letters and requests to psycho-analyse me continued over the following eighteen months, asking the same bizarre psychoanalytical questions.

In light of this strange cumulative behaviour, I requested for certain medical professionals to no longer be involved in my care and asked for them to please stop contacting me.

In other parts of my life, I was also still having to deal with being berated in public where I lived—something that had always happened in the past with some women (the particular aspects of me that had been kindly deemed to be good qualities by others, seemed to prompt these women's abusive behaviour), but had now been taken to a whole new level with them, as I was now in pain as a result of the cancer treatment.

'Just ignore them. They're idiots,' Ethan would tell me.

I thought that with time, such incidences would likely lessen or cease altogether. How very mistaken I was.

Another miserable winter came around. Ethan and I struggled with immense difficulty, due to the circumstances that we were living in, even when it came to providing the bare essentials. We did not have a car or mobile phones. We prioritized the bills and forwent everything in the material and leisure sense to do so.

But what made this situation more depressing, was the knowledge that I should have by now earned a very comfortable standard of living due to having been noticed from a young age for what was apparently felt to be my suitability for the performing arts and writing. Instead, my life took a different route beyond my control, and I was now living in a situation of endless misery and deprivation.

Though, as Ethan worked hard so often, I was alone most of the time at this desolate time in my life, I did not feel lonely. Not only was I was used to isolation through my earlier circumstances of deprivation and then of the misdiagnosis, but also life had made me into a very un-needy person.

There was nothing that I could do but adapt to my circumstances and make the most of my situation with as many of my interests as I could manage while recovering from the cancer treatment and without help or money, including music and reading. But I did feel terribly low at my situation, embarrassed by the circumstances that I found myself in and downhearted that my life was being wasted when I had the potential to do so much with it.

The cancer itself I had always been able to cope with; my young life and all the things that I could do with it being completely wasted however, made me feel intensely, frustratedly sad.

During the winter, the house was very cold once again, meaning those familiar iced-over-on-the-inside windows returned as the snow crept in. In my condition of physical rehabilitation at the time, I continued to struggle with using the very old bathroom, with its frosty breeze permeating the thin window with its rusting frame. Our penurious circumstances, due to the effects of my suffering the cancer symptoms for so long, had left the house quite dull and uncomfortable in its slowly increasing journey towards possible dilapidation and it was in need of repair. Having, by way of my situation, no choice but to spend most of my time in these surroundings for some time to come, however harsh the winters were or however glorious the summers might have been. felt utterly miserable. It was a desolate existence that I longed to get out of.

I did not have any social media, and through deep abashment at anyone knowing about what I was living through, I kept my ordeal entirely secret. Hardly anyone knew that I existed for many years. But you know what? There is absolutely nothing to fear in that regard, and you have to feel comfortable being by yourself — something I have always had ease with my entire life.

But my dire circumstances made life tough. With no means whatsoever of having any lightness in my life and not being able to go anywhere due to lack of money, I was stuck in a deprived and dreary, extremely stressful, painful, and isolated existence for many years.

No matter what I went through however, I never once thought, 'Why me?' I simply accepted that this was the hand that I had been dealt in life and that I had to manage it as best I could to get myself out of it as much as possible.

Earlier in the year, I had discovered two other young women who had also received misread tests over the same period of time and were now being treated for cervical cancer—though on neither count, not to the extent that I was—which had seemed very coincidental and now, I was discovering more of them through a little relevant research. I am limited legally with what I can disclose with regards to other women possibly affected by such matters and how I came to learn about them, but to the best of my knowledge, our misreported tests had all taken place during the same time period. I was informed by someone who had professional knowledge of the situation, that allegedly at least two of those who had misread cervical screening testing had succumbed to the resulting cervical cancer. I had most unnervingly discovered this, but I could not say anything about it.

As the only one of the people affected who had noticed the other possible cases, I now felt a huge responsibility to others with this. It seemed that what I had unwittingly uncovered was something that was not supposed to happen. This was unknown about, other than to a couple of legal professionals or medical staff who had concerns about the issues, and could thus continue, potentially resulting in more young women having their lives destroyed or even lost. So, despite my wretched situation, I put as much effort as I could manage into attempting to piece together the whole situation and see if I could help make things better for others.

This knowledge, my involvement in it, and what I should do about it in regard to pursuing some kind of legal action weighed down on my already-heavy shoulders. But I was told that there was nothing I could do about it apart from, as had been advised, going to the press, and I would not do that as I wanted to maintain my anonymity.

After a couple of years of the vivid nightmares and struggling with my changed life, I overcame my embarrassment about this to briefly mention it to my new, forward-thinking and efficient doctor during one of the check-ups for the cancer treatment complications.

'You are traumatised,' he said simply. 'You have had a huge amount of acute stress to deal with, and I think that, combined with the changes to your body due to the cancer treatment, has caused you to understandably be feeling very down at your situation. I am going to contact a psychology department to get you some physical health therapy.'

I felt that familiar fear again and quietly begged, '*Please* no, I can't go through that again with those people in those areas of the medical field...not the psychoanalyses again...'

'You don't need to worry about that anymore, okay?' he told me reassuringly. 'We know now that they got that wrong. This would not be that kind of psychological therapy; rather, I think you need specialist adjustment therapy for people who have had physical trauma. There is a physical health therapist within the Psychology

Department. I will refer you to them.'

The extent of my medical needs at this time required specialist care and I received treatment from specialists for pain, physiotherapy, and urology in various parts of England. Some of the medics who were now involved in my medical care knew about the lengthy misdiagnosis that had caused my health problems and spoke to me openly about this.

One of them, a leading specialist of his field, upon learning of the misdiagnosis, did not hold back in telling Ethan and I of his disgust about it, which took me by complete surprise. 'I hope that you will pursue legal action,' he told us, with an almost infuriated earnestness. I must have looked taken aback by his response, as he stated just how disgraceful he thought the whole fiasco to have been, and he expressed deep sympathy at what I had endured.

Until now, I had harboured a fear that clinicians would view me with scorn as a result of any upheaval that the effects of the misdiagnosis or the legal matters surrounding it may have caused, but such a worry dissolved at the compassion and understanding I was shown by these wonderful medical professionals. They helped to maintain my trust when having to see clinicians for my ongoing treatment, given my previous experiences in this regard. When I spoke to them about my fears of others knowing about the medical negligence and how I may inadvertently offend some medical professionals by speaking about those experiences, they had been unanimous in their supportive feedback: what had happened to me was wrong, they said, and should not be glossed over.

Despite some of the degrading things that I had previously been subjected to in a clinical setting as a result of the misdiagnosis, that aside, I since received truly conscientious medical care from profoundly competent, skilled and caring clinicians, for which I am incredibly grateful.

The swelling in my lower body since the major surgery, increasingly worsened.

I must admit that I felt sad at the loss of my super-healthy body and particular physique. 'But your body is still beautiful,' said Ethan. 'You still have your shape. You are just swollen because of the effects of the treatment, but it will get better. Your normal figure will return with treatment for the swelling.'

Notably, to correct some of the damage caused by the cancer treatment, it was necessary for me to undergo more lower abdominal surgery. The extraordinarily talented and affable urological surgeon who treated me even managed to completely avoid any requirement for a urostomy by skilfully repairing what he could of my body and I was enormously thankful for ultimately not needing to have that procedure.

However, nothing that even the most highly skilled specialists could do could repair the irreversible painful effects of the cancer treatment.

Over the coming year, I received even more strange letters from the consultant and psychiatrist asking me to attend meetings for the purposes of research, along with the same inappropriate and bizarre psychoanalytical questions. After what I had lived through with being wrongly classed as imagining the symptoms of my cancer, with the opening of each such letter that arrived, my stomach would turn with fear and dread. When would this strangeness with my medical care ever end? *Why can't they just treat me in a straightforward manner and accept the fact that it has been proven that I was a normal-minded individual whose symptoms of cancer had been genuine?* I thought.

During this time, I yearned to re-access the very things that I had always used as tools to manage stress, including dance. I had danced for all of my life—I danced when I was happy; I danced when I was sad—so now not being able to access that, for the foreseeable future at least, was very difficult to manage.

The meeting with the physical health therapist from the psychology department arrived, and I was assigned both a psychologist and therapist to aid in my recovery. I felt embarrassed at accepting this therapy, even though it was only connected to physical health changes but was completely open to it in spite of being in dread of a repeat of what happened in the misdiagnosis and having to go through a similarly horrendous business again. However, it turned out that I need not have worried at all: upon our first meeting, I found the psychologist, Jenny, to be a gentle and understanding woman. She did not probe into my early life but instead focused on the effects of my misdiagnosis and cancer treatment, as well as how I was managing my changed life and body. It was not anything inappropriate, and so I began to relax with these new medical professionals who were helping to correct some of the damage that others in their profession had caused.

My physical health therapist, Laura, was very amiable and straight-talking, I instantly felt comfortable with her: in our first meeting, she had my medical file in front of her, detailing what the psychiatrist had previously said about me: that they believed my pain and bleeding to be psychosomatic as a result of my being from a deprived background, or were possibly (bizarrely, on the sole basis of my slim appearance) attributable to an eating disorder. She read through it thoroughly, along with the information on my misdiagnosis, and, having worked extensively in psychiatry, concluded that, now that my physical symptoms had been proven to be genuine and that I had been shown to not have any behavioural problems or mental illness, the psychiatrist's opinion had simply been speculative and based on typical textbook theory. She threw the file with the psychiatrist's notes to one side and declared, 'Right, let's ignore that load of nonsense!'

After some assessment by Jenny and Laura, I was informed that I was suffering from post-traumatic stress as a result of my experiences in medical care, the prolonged misdiagnosis, and also for my experiences in some of society following this.

Considering the extent of the damage from the cancer treatment and misdiagnosis and the immensity of the impact it had left on me in all areas of my life, Jenny and Laura both provided me with the trauma therapy every couple of weeks for the next twelve months. I did not take antidepressants or any other such medication, and there was no requirement for me to, either.

'Your strong core values are what have got you through everything,' Jenny commented. Later, those very same strong core values would become a source of outright ridicule to at least one particular person.

The verbal abuse in public, almost always by women, continued. Thankfully, this did not happen all the time and it was never from everyone, of course, and some people were lovely to me, but there were enough of the instigators about for it to be a frequent occurrence, usually with them yelling who did I think I was wearing that dress or having that hair, combined with pointing out how the cancer treatment had affected me, such as at the time, the abdominal swelling, being that I was not yet being provided the full treatment needed to control this.

When faced with their jeering comments, or sometimes, aggression, I tried to remain characteristically serene, fighting my natural reaction to lower my head in discomfort at the situation, which was what I had sometimes done before.

'They are idiots, Beck,' Ethan said, 'just ignore them.'

What the women who behaved that way towards me were completely unaware of, besides what I had lived through, was that I had been doing the very best I could privately to bring about improvements to cervical cancer care and preventative care for them and their sisters, friends, and daughters so that they would never experience what I had gone through and would also have a better chance of their lives being saved, should they become ill with cervical cancer. That, and the fact that I had allowed my body and my clinical case to be used for vital research for the very same reasons.

When I came to tell Laura of such experiences, she said, 'That's called "pack mentality": they can sense your vulnerability, despite your best intentions of trying to hide what you have been through, and you also have a lovely, intriguing manner about you and that nice way of carrying yourself. Those women delight in exploiting any weakness they perceive in you in order to make themselves feel better than you. Now you may struggle to understand this, since you don't think like that or have that kind of personality, but that is the way some people are, and these types of people tend to act together in groups because it increases their power; that's what pack mentality is.'

I wondered what I was supposed to do about it: in the past, I had tried to placate them by almost changing myself to try and fit in, but that had been soul-destroying for me. 'You don't have to do anything', Laura said, 'Their behaviour speaks volumes about who they are. Those women were jealous of you'.

It was very difficult to comprehend why anyone would feel the way that Laura had described, and I would never assume that anyone would. If that truly was the case as I was being told, then there was absolutely no reason at all for it as far as I was concerned and it felt sort of embarrassing. I wondered if the instigators would feel differently had they known how my life had been.

Laura added, 'if those women had even a quarter of the pain you live with each day, they would think that they were dying', with her reasoning that they were weak-minded. All I knew was that I was heartily tired of having to deal with them. But I took comfort in the fact that many others did not treat me that way and were so nice to me.

Sharing with Laura that I worried I might possibly have something wrong with my mind or some kind of flaw that I was not aware of and needed correcting, after what I had been told about people from a background who had suffered deprivation and abuse, she responded with a warm smile, 'What you perhaps don't realise is that both Jenny and I have analysed you and your life just as a routine part of the job that we do and let me assure you that, having done that and seeing your home life often, there is absolutely nothing like that about you at all. You are traumatised by your experiences surrounding the misdiagnosis and the way you have been treated since, but that's totally understandable, and I have great belief that you are strong enough to get through that. You must understand that this has been wrongly put into your mind by others, and now, we have to try and *undo* it. Some people have made you feel *terrible* about yourself. But I *have* noticed something distinctive about your character, Beck—and it's not a bad thing. You are an empathetic person'. She continued 'But your empathetic nature combined with how you have been groomed to think that your personal boundaries don't matter means that you can be taken advantage of'.'

Where empathy is concerned, I feel that strong instinctive feeling is a part of oneself that is acted on without actually giving any thought to it. I mean, we process the *feelings* of empathy and deeply internalise them, but we don't intellectualise over this, instead only experiencing that this powerful natural pull that we feel to the very core of ourself is indicative of the most humane thing: an urge to act in accordance of decency with at any given moment; something tangible, a deep understanding and intuition of pain or discomfort and that gut-wrenching intense feeling of finding witnessing suffering, whether of human or animal, unbearable.

So, in this respect, I hadn't properly considered that others might misuse my empathetic type of nature and that it had at times been exploited. When Laura explained to me that this, and my circumstances, had so far made me susceptible to manipulative behaviours from some, I learned that it was imperative for me to develop stronger boundaries, in order to protect myself from the possibilities of being abusively preyed on in the future.

The thing is, I had often tried to stand up for myself when it was apparent that I needed to, but I was either taken no notice of or would be told that I was wrong to respond, and I had therefore felt powerless to do anything about it, particularly as some made a point of telling me, subtly or otherwise, how I was obligated to do as they said for those very reasons. Other times, I had allowed people to do this so as simply not to have to endure their rage or threats. But for the most part, I hadn't even fully comprehended at the time what exactly was being done to me, for as I learned, I had been conditioned that way.

But now I was becoming aware that the unfortunate circumstances of my life thus far had put me in the position of someone who could be abused. I knew that I did not want to live the rest of my life like that and that I had to make changes to it, but I had no idea how to—and yet I knew that I must.

My strange and unpleasant life experiences increased as more information surrounding aspects of my misdiagnosis was revealed— and, ultimately, it transpired that if it were not for the interference of some in psychiatry and psychology, the departments of which had never been a part of my life until I developed the tumour, along with the tests being misread, my tumour symptoms would have been taken seriously and I would have been diagnosed *before* reaching the stage of requiring life-changing treatment. Those who had defined my pain and bleeding as psychosomatic and had consequently wrongly referred me for psychological assessment now continually cited in their defence that they were simply entirely influenced by the negative test results. Indeed, that was the sole reason given for the psychiatrist coming to see me at all in the first instance all those years earlier, while I was in hospital with the physical symptoms.

It was also explained to me by a professional of psychology that what had happened to me with the misdiagnosis had been not that uncommon an experience in the past, whereby some young women—especially ones who may have been fascinating or seen as having some kind of appeal in some way—had been subjected to unnecessary psychiatric evaluation or even treatment, for reasons that were not legitimate and could not be clinically proven. Such horrors were unspoken of then, hidden away in files and behind closed doors (though I am not comparing those horrendous experiences to what happened to me in the misdiagnosis).

I worried that, if others were to ever find out that I may have been something of the modern-day version of this, that they would possibly entirely miss the point that in fact, I had been fundamentally misdiagnosed—so I did not reveal what I had lived through to anyone for a long time indeed.

I was also later told by a very competent psychology professional that the conclusion of 'psychosomatic pain and bleeding due to possible depression' might have allowed some of those involved in my medical care to skirt around the fact that they had not found me to have any mental illness but still allowed them to analyse me for whatever purpose suited them, whether out of inappropriate curiosity or attempts to prove theory. 'Even though you were not found to be terribly damaged from your early years or to have any mental illness, the incorrect cervical screening results gave them reason to analyse you when there should have been no reason to at all', they said. In this respect, I recalled some of the bizarre and sometimes inappropriate questions they had sometimes asked me, including about my body and appearance. Among the comments that were made in this respect, were, when explaining to one medical professional how the pain and bleeding symptoms were impacting my ability to work consistently and thereby leading me into a spiral of poverty, 'Well, with how you look, getting on in life shouldn't be a problem for you'.

In the midst of the legal process, some of those involved chose to place further pressure on my shoulders when Ethan required surgery, for which he was recovering for a few months. Some were blatantly smug and callous about putting me through the mill as much as possible. When they couldn't find anything in my behaviour to use against me, it was demeaning that they frequently cited my impoverished, neglectful and abused teen years as reasons for me not be a person worthy of any consideration or help. 'Someone from her background would never have become anything anyway' one said.

Those responsible for my being in this situation did not seem to think that their admission of errors carried much weight, as instead, some of their representatives took the measure of looking for any way that they could to try and blame me for the effects of the misdiagnosis and misread testing.

This included subjecting me to further psychological evaluation.

A psychiatrist went to town on focusing (again) solely on my deprived early years, believing that this is what entirely defines a person (thankfully, this theoretical and blanket view towards those who have experienced deprivation and abuse in their early lives, however very individual a person might be, seems not to be one shared by all professionals of the health of the mind), completely ignoring all the things in my life that suggested that there might be some chance of me being perhaps a balanced adult. At the same time, that which I experienced at the hands of their colleagues during the misdiagnosis was not acknowledged in any way, and when I politely tried to talk about it and how it had impacted my life, they simply ignored me.

Astoundingly, someone who psychologically evaluated me for the purposes of possible legal proceedings relating to the negligence in my medical care, at first said that they agreed with the original opinion of the psychiatrist—the pain and bleeding being psychosomatic—until it was explained to them, perhaps embarrassingly for their part, that this theory had been outrightly disproven by the historical diagnosis of the cancer and the fact that my reporting of my symptoms had exactly coincided with the dates of all the incorrect tests. Ultimately, because of this, they very reluctantly admitted that the opinion of those who had misdiagnosed me had been incorrect—an opinion that, once it had been stated, was taken almost as gospel and influenced almost everything else that happened with my medical care. But they were begrudging about this; instead of humbly learning from the mistake borne of incorrect theory, they seemed disgruntled that an opinion of anyone of their profession had been questioned and found to be wrong.

While one psychiatrist noted, 'all credit to her, she has overcome everything she has gone through in life very well,' I was perplexed to find they could not let go of my deprived early years, as much of the theory of the profession seems fixated on searching for anything in a person that could deem them to be damaged from their early lives.

One of the intentions for this, seemed to be to try and place the blame for the misdiagnosis on anything other than that which anyone involved in my medical care might have done. But also, there was a fascination by some of how, coming from my background, I had developed as an adult and not turned out the way that much of the theory states. This attitude once again fuelled that dreaded feeling that I might forever be judged on having an unfortunate start in life, rather than the person that I had become, and that people would want to go over it all again and again and again.

As previously, I was asked multiple times; *how do you react to stress? How do you cope with stress?* Having been asked this many times over the years and now having to answer this again during these additional analyses really wore me down. Nevertheless, I politely answered that given that I was not an angry person, had never had any addictions, had never taken antidepressants, had never gone around breaking the law or hurting people in any way, tried (I hope) to be as considerate as possible towards others, and that I was trying my best to live my life as healthily, calmly, and in as civilized a way as possible despite everything I had lived through, I was therefore surely, logically, fairly okay at managing stress.

But they still seemed to want to see how I would react under pressure, not comprehending that I had in fact been living with extreme stress for most of my life due to circumstance and was in fact, continuing to do so acutely at that moment.

Their frustration at having analysed every part of my life and having not found me to be the way that some of the traditional theory suggests that a person of my deprived early life might be, was almost tangible. I was almost repeatedly made to explain for it, with the degradation of an analysis seemingly into almost every aspect of who I was and what I had experienced, They could not separate that in order to see me for the individual that I was. 'How is this possible', they queried, after every area of my life was scrutinized, 'for her not to have any addictions, no trouble with the law whatsoever, no chaotic life, no mental illness, nothing at all of note'.

'If I may humbly offer an insight,' I politely and gently responded, 'there are various elements that attribute to my values and outlook on life. But what *is* possible is that maybe Freudian theoretical textbook thinking regarding our early lives is not so accurate after all—at least in the case of those like me.'

There is in fact no great mystery to it: I simply always had a strong urge to overcome adversity and, along with this, due to my type of nature, had a desire to live my life in an unchaotic manner, and hopefully make something good of it, was always willing to take personal responsibility for myself and also, crucially, to be considerate of others (I do not believe that anything from our early lives forms reason to treat others badly in any way). Actually, often those who have suffered greatly in their lives are deeply compassionate people, because you know that pain well, to the very heart of you, and you don't want others to experience it.

None of these particular professionals of the mind had at all recognised that there was of course something of note by way of my being affected by my early years and most significantly so, but it presented itself differently to that of some of the textbook expectations of some parts of psychiatry of what someone from my type of background should apparently become. The way I *had* been affected by my early years, definitively by my adolescence, was that I would put the needs of others before myself apparently too much, often diminish myself to placate others and believe others' voice, opinions, and wellbeing to matter more than mine. What they also missed was that what had happened to me during the misdiagnosis had compounded this further.

It ultimately took some gentle persuasion from Laura before I finally confided to her the full extent of what happened in the misdiagnosis and after the radical surgery. To my surprise, she became silent and slightly tearful upon hearing my descriptions of what I had experienced. Until then, I felt that I had simply been feeling sorry for myself, but I now realised that there had perhaps been a bit of something valid in my being affected by what I had been subjected to.

The trauma I experienced, so I was told, had all the features of someone who has been tortured, and apparently, by definition, that is what had happened to me. That was the very approach that was taken to manage it, especially for the nightmares and the effects of people's repeated questioning and the circumstances that I had managed for so long. Now, during these sessions, my trauma was sensibly viewed simply as a natural response to what I had been through.

I was advised that, in light of the misdiagnosis now being official, though medical records can never be changed, a note could be added, stating that there were no psychological issues noted prior to my reporting the symptoms of the cancer, and that it had been merely an opinion at the time based entirely on the incorrect screening test results and that this opinion had since been disproven by the confirmation of my historic cervical cancer and the subsequent misdiagnosis.

Finally, I was officially free of the stigma of the incompetent opinion of those who had caused the misdiagnosis; albeit by now, sixteen years too late. The doctors involved in my medical care no longer took any notice whatsoever of the opinions of those who had misdiagnosed me. To my absolute relief, none of that would be part of my life anymore and I would be treated completely normally by medical professionals from now on.

But all of the damage that had been done as a result of the misdiagnosis could not be erased or corrected, and I would have to live with it forever.

More revelations concerning the errors with my medical care were uncovered, including a personally disconcerting one that even further heightened my feelings of discomfort at the unusual circumstances of my life: I was informed that I was the most badly affected survivor of what seemed to be, as I had suspected and tried to raise the issue of, some others who had misread cervical screening tests: my misdiagnosis had been the lengthiest, and the physical effects of it the most severe.

I had also been the only one who had been repeatedly psychologically analysed. The reason for this, seemed to be attributable partly to the symptoms that I had, given that I developed a high-grade tumour, situated deep inside the cervix so the pain and bleeding might have been a bit more troublesome, leading me to repeatedly report it, and because, when I did so, the testing at the time was stated as not showing any gynaecological problems, that assessment was ordered to determine if the symptoms were psychological. With psychological analyses focused on one's early years as standard, and with the discovery that my adolescence had been so deprived and abusive, that was then immediately seized on as the apparent reason why I was supposedly imagining the gynaecological symptoms, with them being deemed 'psychosomatic gynaecological symptoms possibly due to depression.'

So now, I found myself in the very solitary and strange position of being not only the survivor who had unwittingly uncovered the possibility of other cases and a wider picture of something being terribly wrong with the cervical screening procedures at that time, but also the one who was the worst affected by way of my misdiagnosis and the resulting treatment. This all made for a difficult position to bear, weighing down heavily on me—and it was one that I managed in silence for many years.

Despite the medical establishment's admission of incompetence in allowing me to develop cancer, it was an unpleasant and lengthy battle to get any actual explanation from them as to why this had happened or to try to do anything about it legally.

Some insightful experts who were participating in the legal matters had warned those involved of my lack of quality of life and urged them to consider that. However, their opinions did not seem to have been taken seriously; others continued to act in accordance with their unfounded beliefs, even initially stating that the diagnosed lymphoedema that I had developed as a result of the treatment for the cancer, was delusional—and, when it became indisputable that I did have the illness, they then implied that that I was somehow to blame for the health problems that I had as a result of the cancer treatment and that they did not really affect me. It was as though I was repeating those twelve years all over again—but now, it was intensely worse.

Although it was shown that the opinions of those within the misdiagnosis had been very mistaken indeed, those trying to defend their actions still did not seem to care.

The unscrupulous tactics that some continued to use, made it very easy for them to try to break me as a person with their ways of defining matters. A strategy, so I was informed, often used in this type of situation, making it feel as though it is the affected individual who is at fault in one way or another, despite there being solid evidence that they are suffering so severely as a result of someone else's actions. But however exasperating and hurtful that was, I was not the first and I will not be the last as a person who has had something ghastly brought upon them, to be subjected to that particular cruelness of the legal-procedure arena.

This course of action was not what I would ever have liked to have decided on; I felt uneasy about being blameful towards people by taking this route, as I have absolute respect for the healthcare in England and for the medical professionals who work within it. But although I did not want to cause upheaval to anyone, the dreadful circumstances that I had been left in and the questions surrounding the prolonged misdiagnosis and the cervical screening issues, suggested that this procedure was both very much needed and appropriate. However, I found the whole process to be profoundly stressful and often undignified.

In my adolescence and at times in my young adult life, if I had dared to politely speak up for myself or gently articulate that I was being caused distress, I would aggressively be told 'Shut. Up.' With fear, I would always comply. Now, I was facing a similar scenario here: though not literally told to shut up in this case, any attempt to politely convey the extent of my pain or how I had been affected by the experiences of the misdiagnosis was often quashed immediately, without being given a chance to properly speak.

Eventually, I was informed that, despite their very significant role in my cancer being missed, the psychiatry and psychology professionals could simply cite the incorrect cervical screening test results as the cause of their misdiagnosis and consequent unnecessary psychological analyses. This would, in turn, leave them devoid of responsibility. This also applied to the doctor who had relied on the incorrect test results and the psychiatrist's opinion. 'It was the test results being wrong that are at fault, not us' was the reason constantly used to pass the blame for what had happened to me.

But the reasons behind what had happened with the testing remained unclear and nobody seemed to be being held accountable for those either.

It seems that those responsible for taking my life down an excruciating, frightening, and deprived path might have been blinded by their own certainty that their theory must be correct or simply have seen me as interesting for their work—and there is the distinct possibility that they could have stopped my suffering in its tracks, but for reasons that would not be known, they chose not to. They declined to tell me anything about how medical ethics or procedure had been managed (later, I would come to realise that it would not be helpful for me to know; it served no purpose for my wellbeing).

In the end, the establishment responsible for the misdiagnosis and screening tests ultimately lost in the legal action that was brought against them, and I won (and I was grateful to those affable and skilled professionals who helped me in the legal procedure).

But despite that fact, and the pain that I had suffered for all of those years had been proven to be due to my living with a cancerous tumour all along, this was a hollow victory for me. Though I was thankful for any help that I was given, much of that which I needed to rebuild my life and take care of myself for the rest of my life with my health problems as a result of the cancer treatment would not be made available to me, as well as being informed that I could not take legal action against those medical professionals responsible for the damage to my life, as they were able to simply blame the incorrect cervical screening tests by stating that it was only their opinion at the time based on those incorrect tests (and for some of those involved, I do in fact feel compassion for that statement as it may genuinely have been the case that they were completely ignorant to the fact that I had developed cancer).

Unfortunately, that is just the way it goes with these matters sometimes; an optimal outcome is not guaranteed for anyone, even when one has won, as I did. As difficult as it was, I had to accept this and let it go.

But the shattering reality of what I was facing set in. Nothing could give me back all those years of my young life that I had lost, that by now amounted to almost two decades—the very years that were supposed to shape a life of accomplishment that I had been trying to build and work towards.

Although it was brightness and tranquillity that I craved, the all-consuming sadness that I felt permeated my daily reality. I was now left facing a very bleak future indeed.

Though I tried not to feel sorry for myself, I had effectively been told that my life was over, and it absolutely seemed that way. How would I ever rebuild it now?

13
Pretty Outcast

I T WAS THE AUTUMN OF 2015, and my life, future, and whole sense of self had been almost shattered. Curiously, I still loved life, and yet I did not feel that I had any place in it.

The effect of my life experiences slowly but surely became completely soul-destroying.

Despite my depressing circumstances and pain, there was some light; the course of the small mortgage on our home had now reached completion, having forgone so much to commit to paying it off, and the property had tripled in value during that time. The penury that Ethan and I had lived in for years finally resolved, as we continued to make sensible financial decisions.

Some travel was therefore now financially feasible again and we took our first holiday in years. I had been informed about the effects of air travel on lymphoedema and knew that flights would cause further swelling, though only temporarily, and was taught how to manage with this. Having been advised to only fly a short distance while I got used to managing the effects that flying has on lymphoedema,

Though I was uncomfortable at first in managing my health conditions for the first time while returning to travelling, I loved the feel of the sun and sand again; of touching palm trees and looking at colourful flowers, always focusing on the fabulous parts of life.

However, my distended abdomen worsened, along with pain in my legs. I maintained the gait and posture that I previously had, but it was difficult to do so, given the pain that I was constantly in.

Constant treatment would have brought the swelling under control, but for now, it was reaching levels that were further impeding on my chances of having any quality of life.

The bit of therapy for the trauma and physical health adjustment had run its course and came to an end. 'Your resilience is *amazing*,' said Laura.

That was a kind thing to say, but really I had known for most of my life that I had no choice but to accept the hand that I had been dealt and get on with things.

Laura added that she knew that I just wanted to get on with my life and make something good of it, and that was so true.

I told her however that I still had those worries about myself as somehow being defective because of the circumstances of my beginnings and what I had lived through since with the misdiagnosis. But Laura reiterated, 'Those people have done a *real* number on you', she responded sombrely. 'They have not only ruined your life, but they have almost totally destroyed your sense of self-perception'. I was surprised at her seriousness as I listened to her earnestly tell me, 'You have been wrongly made to feel that way about yourself. There's *absolutely nothing* wrong with you like that, Beck. You are a stable-minded person. Your type of trauma from the misdiagnosis and the abuse that you were subjected to as an effect of that will resolve to be manageable in time. I think you're actually going to go on to do really well in life.' Hearing those words from a pragmatic expert of the mind reassured me, and to learn from a few other medical professionals, including some in psychology, that I was ultimately declared absolutely fine in that regard, was a relief.

The lymphoedema (not to be confused with lipoedema which is a completely different condition and which I do not have) continued to progress into more and more of a problem—and it was not showing any sign of letting up: my formerly strong dancer legs and defined abdomen were now swollen, and I felt so embarrassed at this. I was yet to receive the necessary properly customised treatment for the illness at this point.

I pushed myself to continue to walk and be active but was in constant pain and learning to adapt to my legs and feet not having the full feeling that they had previously.

Lymphoedema specialists oftentimes describe the effect of the illness with this helpful analogy: 'The removal of the lymph nodes results in an effect like a dripping tap; you can drain the bath, but it will quickly fill up again.' Therefore, dealing with this takes daily maintenance.

As time went on, Ethan grew more concerned about the lymphoedema worsening and so spoke to specialists about this. We were informed of the possibility of more intensive treatment in other parts of the world, as treatment is limited in the UK.

A few months later, I was booked into a lymphoedema hospital in Austria.

When we arrived there, I was very physically uncomfortable and looked ill, with swelling to my abdomen and legs that felt incredibly tender.

Due to my having had so many of my lymphatic nodes—essentially the pumping mechanism for the lymphatic system—removed in my pelvic and groin areas, the only way that the lymphatic fluid in my legs and pelvis could move was if it was manually stimulated into doing so via intense lymphatic drainage massage. Hence, the hospital would focus on this, alongside other supporting therapies, including compression.

Lymphatic drainage has become popular for 'pampering' or helping to remove toxins from the body. However, in a lymphatically healthy body, while it can be helpful, lymphatic drainage is not a necessity. I personally find it strange to hear people who have lymphatically healthy bodies complaining about 'needing' lymphatic drainage. I can only assume that it is due to an uneducated misconception of some of how the lymphatic system functions. In my case, however, with such a heavily compromised lymph system, lymphatic drainage is essential in the prevention of becoming seriously unwell.

When the specialist doctor at the hospital first examined me, she found that the situation was worse than we had known. She looked at Ethan with shock upon her findings, explaining to him how severe a problem there was, including her concern over the lymphorrhagia that I initially suffered after my surgery.

She also found that I had high arterial pressure in my legs at the time—something that can apparently be caused by the knock-on effects of the pressure of the disrupted lymph fluid flow. I was clearly in a very bad way.

Any hope that I had previously held concerning an almost complete recovery faded as soon as I had the full diagnosis on the lymphoedema: this was my life now, and I had to accept it. I had always had every intention of doing so, of course, but I never realised just how very severely the misdiagnosis and cancer treatment had affected me until now.

The treatment schedule devised for me was intense, with drainage and bandaging sessions all day.

People from all over the world came for treatment at the hospital. Many were very friendly and some also very humorous.

But my adjustment problems in adapting to the lymphoedema were compounded by the intense treatment. I loathed the whole thing. I had great difficulty with accepting that I had to wear the compression alternately, imperatively so when exercising and taking any flight. I could not explain the way that I felt about this; I just remained very quiet and kept it to myself.

One hot summer's day there, Ethan and I wanted to go out walking. Without a cloud in the blue sky, the weather, along with the stunning natural surroundings of the alps and greenery, made for relaxing viewing—the exact type of leisurely thing I normally love to experience. However, on this occasion, I was hesitant to go anywhere because of feeling so psychologically uncomfortable at the lymphoedema and the treatment for it.

But Ethan told me, 'It will be fine; just focus on having a nice afternoon.'

Hence, I coached myself in my mind to face my embarrassment, and, with that, we set off slowly into the town, me linking his arm. Ethan found a cute little café and pulled up a chair for me in the shade of a canopy at one of the outside tables. The people at the café were kind to me, and one lady, who spoke excellent English, became a little choked up after enquiring to Ethan about my health. 'Aww, so sad, a girl like that', she said. I was stunned at being shown such empathy.

The doctor arranged counselling sessions with her and the

hospital's psychologist. Initially I was afraid of this, given my previous experiences of being unnecessarily analysed when I had reported the cancer symptoms—but I needn't have worried, as they were both very sensible and intuitive in their work, never once mentioning unfounded theoretical rhetoric and with, thankfully, no interest whatsoever in my formative and adolescent years.

'This is devastating for a young woman like you,' the doctor said firmly, 'But you have survived and should use everything that is good about yourself to get a good life.'

The lead doctor and psychologists' therapy sessions helped with my feelings of embarrassment at the circumstances I had lived through and the effects of this. 'All of that emotion you have stored inside, you need to let out,' said the psychologist, 'It is not healthy for you to be expected to continue like nothing has happened to you or deny how bad what you have been through is, and you will go through stages with this until you eventually come to accept it.' My way of dealing with the daunting and painful experiences throughout my life has always been to do two things—to accomplish and be cheerful—but never, *never*, my dear, to wallow in the problem—until now. I did not belong anywhere: I was so ashamed of the course that my life had taken, and I had no future, in spite of my best efforts to do something good with my life. These deep feelings of despair had accumulated over time, and now, with the odds so very stacked against me in terms of my ever being able to have some kind of good quality of life, let alone progress with my work as a creative, I could no longer deny them.

Physically however, I began to dramatically improve with the specialised treatment. The lymphoedema immediately began to respond to the days of intensive therapies, and the very skilled therapists could feel this positive response as they treated me, my true physique slowly beginning to show through under the affected areas. I had arrived at the hospital looking pale and completely exhausted, but now, I looked so much healthier. 'Getting stronger,' said a lymphatic masseuse proudly, who had been putting much effort into treating me (lymphoedema treatment can be hard physical work for those issuing it)—and he was right: the treatment and knowledge of the staff here, combined with the peaceful environment, was helping me to recover. I did, however, still have a way to go with the adjustment side of things.

After a few weeks, I was out of the danger zone of becoming severely ill with lymphoedema. Hence, with a rigid treatment plan in place, I was able to exercise properly once again, and I could return home.

Back in the UK, though the swelling had been very much reduced and was now becoming undetectable, I now had to continue the lymphoedema treatment for the rest of my life in order to keep it that way. Eventually, I would receive conscientious medical care for this from some caring Lymphoedema nurses who were excellent in their work.

Exercise is also one of the crucial parts of the everyday treatment for lymphoedema, as staying active is essential to managing the illness in that this stimulates the lymphatic system, and I was keen to continue to be as athletic as possible anyway. Apart from dance, something active that I had missed throughout my treatment was cycling. Before my illness, I had always cycled most days, partly because of the sense of freedom that it gave me. Because of the effects of the cancer treatment, however, I had not been able to get back on a bike for the past six years, but now, because I had been helped so much to regain my fitness at the lymphoedema hospital, Ethan felt I may be ready to begin cycling again and he found me a stylish vintage bike which would be comfortable enough for my health conditions. Henceforth, I cycled regularly again, including to and from the places that provided my medical treatment. It took every inch of my physical and mental endurance to do so sometimes; it was terribly harsh to do this in the middle of winter, in freezing weather conditions, and with my health problems, and was always painful, but I carried on regardless.

As I attempted to navigate my way through my changed life, now once more being able to cycle to places where there were fields and flowers, I again sought solace in nature. Being amongst the beauty of nature provides me with happiness and comfort.

Although my cycling again and being back in nature more certainly helped me to manage stress, other areas of my life were still extremely difficult.

Some, when learning that I had told (with reluctance and only when necessary) someone that I was recovering from cancer, would smirkingly question me, 'So *what* type of cancer did you have?' and I would dread having to answer because I knew that upon saying 'cervical', they would either reply with, 'no you haven't' or 'it's your own fault for not going for your smear tests'. I would then have to explain that in fact, I attended them all and had never missed a single one, but they were all not correctly read (I did not tell them however, about having not been believed for twelve years regarding the symptoms), which would then result in a ridiculing response of how, in their minds, that could not possibly be true.

If their ignorance cannot handle the facts about that matter, what would people think about the rest of what I have lived through? I wondered in fear and dreaded having to explain to anyone anything about myself because of such reactions.

Other times when somebody engaged me in friendly conversation, they would swiftly never speak to me again after learning a little of my physical illness, whilst a couple of those who reacted with anger as a result of their concluding my illness not to be real for what they deemed to be fabrication of the cancer (on separate occasions, it was screamed at me, 'you have *not* had cancer') and shouting, in the worst possible terms, about how terrible they thought me to be for that, physically lashed out at me—the worse encounter of the two, as this created a public scene.

Not knowing what to do in these situations, I would always try to ignore the instigators when it became obvious that speaking to them in a civilised way would have no effect. Some of these occasions would embarrassingly leave me a little depressed, shaken, or sometimes mildly tearful.

But I found more and more that my particular case of cancer and also the lymphoedema was something that most people knew nothing about. I did not mind this: I never expected people to understand. Why should they? They were certainly not obliged to. However, while occasionally people were very kind to me about it when they came to learn just a tiny fraction of my having had cancer treatment, let alone the highly unusual experiences surrounding it, many others were blatant and disdainful in their lack of knowledge but with them thinking that they knew it all—some of this was centred on my reserved nature, but also the way that I looked; *you can't have had cancer and yet look so healthy*, was their general train of thought.

I found that some could not grasp that occasionally, some cancers are not at all treatable with chemotherapy, especially those of high-grade like mine, and so not every patient has chemo and instead, radical surgery, as in my case, is the only way to treat the cancer. Having never undergone chemotherapy, I did not lose my hair. Because of my very long hair and healthy-looking appearance, this seemed to prompt some people to say that I did not look ill; this comment not being delivered as a compliment but instead directed with absolute aggressive suspicion. As always, I did not fit in with a stereotype, and so therefore, apparently, there could only be one reason why, in the minds of some with no understanding of such things: it simply was not possible.

Because of this, it was sometimes directly demanded of me to provide evidence of my illness (and always by women). Such matter is plentiful of course but it seemed that they would never understand, regardless of this.

It was strange and contradictory to leave the house and be told spontaneously by some, 'You look lovely,' but, as was more frequently the case, by women in gangs or twos, the usual openly hostile comments over my appearance, accompanied by ridicule at the physical pain that I was in at that time, which was quite apparent from how visibly uncomfortable I was.

Because of this, I became increasingly withdrawn and felt so bad about myself and the way that my life had gone, despite my best efforts to really make a success of it.

An overwhelming sadness enveloped me. I had always been a problem-solver; a logically minded person who could always see ways to adapt to anything. You just plough on through and get on with it. But now, I could see no way ahead if I was being prevented from doing anything with my life.

I struggled to find any sense of self. My entire future had been effectively written off, and, so, though I searched constantly for some meaning to my life, I now could not really find any, no matter how much I tried.

Solely due to circumstance, I had been subjected to abuse, one way or another, for much of my life (something that I had not realised until it was pointed out to me by others) and had lived in hope that at some point, it would stop—but it was becoming more apparent that because of my situation, this would not be so.

This life of trying to manage with three different sources of physical pain as a result of the cancer treatment; of trying to cope with the verbal abuse from the ill-informed people who questioned me over my illness or who expressed anger at my style of clothes, hair, voice or look, of having near-constant insomnia, or, when I did fall asleep, waking up in the night with vivid nightmares of being back in the medical building where I had the extensive surgery; of feeling a guilty sense of not doing enough—at least by societal expectation of such things—to have helped others in the possible cervical screening cases; of not knowing how on Earth I was ever going to progress, or even achieve any better quality of life, was overwhelming. As much as I tried with all my heart and soul, I could no longer see a way out of my situation and of never seeming able to properly protect myself or being able to break-free of the circumstances that prevented me from achieving anything that I was meant to do as a creative, no matter how much effort I put into life and however highly motivated I was.

What was the point, I wondered, *in surviving the misdiagnosis, cancer and the radical treatment for it, if this is the life that I am now facing?*

On some level, at this time, I felt worthless.

The intensely shameful feeling of the often-degrading life that I had lived, weighed down on me. Throughout my life, but especially in recent years on many occasions during the misdiagnosis, cancer treatment and the disturbing events surrounding it, I had been subjected to every indignity, leaving me feeling that I could take no more. I felt forced into an extreme measure that I kept entirely to myself.

I had previously overheard a conversation in a medical setting about medical centres abroad that offered the clinically assisted 'way out' —one of the ultimate dark and depressing subjects and something that I never thought I would find myself ever even being interested in knowing about. Since I had physical issues due to the cancer treatment which resulted in daily pain, this was something that might be an option for me and so, I looked them up. It felt like an immensely strange thing to do as I have always loved life no matter how difficult it might be, but there I was, finding myself reading through all the details.

This was incredibly out of character for me, especially as I had so far faced everything just by getting on with things.

I mulled over this heavy feeling and came to what I felt to be the definitive conclusion: that I could not go on with this life anymore.

Nobody ever knew of these thoughts or plans, as I did not tell a soul—not even Ethan. I doubt I would ever have considered not being here anymore by any other method and I had never felt this way or had any thoughts along those lines before, nor would I since. But this method—a clinical act—felt like my only option. I truly could not see a future for myself anymore.

It was not a decision made on a whim: it was very carefully considered over some time, and I began to make steps to get my affairs in order and begin the process of applying for this end to my life.

I could not have been any more serious about it when one day, something odd happened: I discovered a video link to the process that I was planning to go ahead with. I watched. I wish I never had, frankly; I was personally disturbed by what I saw—and I changed my mind over the whole matter in an instant. (Others' choices or opinions about such things are up to them, but for me personally, it is so that the subject is simply not something that interests me at all).

For me, this had been perhaps a wake-up call: sure, I felt very depressed about my life, I had frequently experienced some kind of abuse throughout almost the entirety of it, and now seemed to have no future prospects whatsoever—but, ultimately, I didn't want to die, and I knew, deep down, that I still had so much to offer life too. It had been something of a 'blip' in my life, a sort of moment of giving in to my circumstances and was an extremely uncomfortable, strange, and out of character place for me to be and one that I would not revisit. *What was I thinking, even considering doing that?* I would later reflect, as I considered how much I appreciated my life. There have after all, been some who never had choice in this matter.

Looking back on this time a few years later, I would find it disturbing to think that I had seriously considered taking such a drastic measure, especially as everything sort of wonderful that I felt in my heart and soul for life and what I could do within it was there then, even though at the time hidden by despair, and could properly begin to later come to the fore, especially in my creativity.

Even if we are in the depths of sadness that feels draining, inescapable and all-consuming: we can go on. Even in some kind of depressing circumstance, we never know how different our lives could be in a year (or months, even) from now; how much better life can get and what wonderful things might be coming our way, even when we least expect them to.

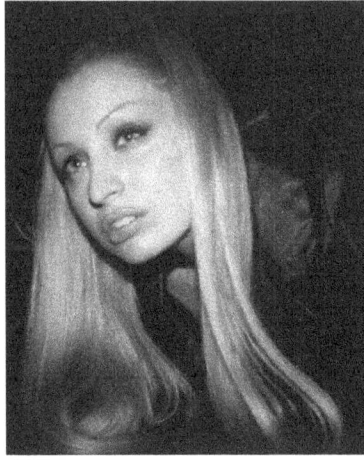

Casting for screen

Photo Credit: R.B.B.

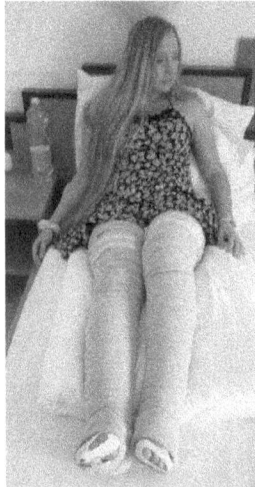

During treatment at the lymphoedema hospital. A low point in my life and I could not look at the camera. (The heavily padded treatment makes my legs look much bigger in the photo than they really are). I have never shown any images of the effects of my illness or treatment before.

Photo Credit: Rebecka Eden-Bond (Private collection)

14
Lost

HAVING CHOSEN TO LIVE MY life—however painful that life may be—I knew that I had to find a way, somehow, of overcoming the particular circumstances that I was in.

By now, I had overcome the trauma to the point of now being able to live with it successfully. In my case, I felt the trauma physically; some things in this regard occasionally gave me a feeling of absolute dread in the pit of my stomach: something that would never go away fully in future, and my body's nervous system had become very reactive over the years due to the fear and extreme stress that I had often been placed under. An additional very troublesome effect of the trauma was generally being unable to sleep no matter how exhausted I would be; I would try to clear my mind but would often have nightmares and feel troubled by some of the abusive experiences surrounding the misdiagnosis, experiences in the place where I had received the cancer treatment and some of those in society, when trying to sleep.

It is my nature to focus on the pleasant; the uplifting; the nice parts of life; but it was not simply a positive mindset that was required here. My life had been almost completely wasted so far, by what had happened to me, and now, I felt completely driven to do something purposeful with it, perhaps more than ever. I began to feel much better about myself too.

Throughout the misdiagnosis and treatment for the effects of the cancer, I had held onto the hope that one day, I would finally have the chance to progress with the creativity, in the performance sense or with my writing, that was kindly spotted in me from a young age.

Despite being encouraged to speak and write publicly by some, I had not only never had the platform necessary to do so, but I also did not feel I had any right to do that; to me, surely nobody would be interested in what I think.

A psychologist had told me that I was living proof that how I had dealt with many difficulties in life, specifically in terms of resilience and mindset, was effective.

But besides that, I very much realised that I had not been at all great with some other areas, such as not setting my own personal boundaries to prevent others from taking advantage of me, struggling to say no to others demands and not prioritising my own wellbeing in situations where that is needed. I am conscious of both my strengths and weaknesses and there is always room for improvement.

Several medical professionals felt that I had dealt with adversity healthily, with one of them explaining to me that I should publicly speak and write about this.

Despite such generous comments however, I gladly leave matters of psychology to the excellent competent experts in that professional field, and of whom there are many brilliant ones.

Rather, I want to put any pinch of knowledge that I might have in relation to the complexity of life (though I do not consider myself at all enlightened in that respect and it is a constant learning process), into my writing or as a performer.

Though it had been suggested to me that I should publicly write and speak in a 'motivational' style due to my experience, my voice style and some of the ways in which I had overcome my experiences, it was not really at all the motivational stuff that I wanted to do; it was to return to becoming a professional creative—except now, I found that with my life experiences, I could put so much more dimension into it.

Indeed, I absolutely wanted to go back to where I had been in the beginning, as my tumour symptoms began, when I had been repeatedly encouraged by the professionals within the arts to develop my work as a creative, but unfortunate circumstances had meant that I had never properly been able to do so. This was a world that I could really lose myself in and where I had always seemed to fit naturally.

As I submitted a couple of film concepts to the production companies, I never really expected a reply, but I was stunned to find that my writing was well-received by some of the small number of those I had forwarded it to.

'I love this! Great title!,' was one such instance of feedback.

But having been asked to forward several months of work showcasing the full concept, when it came to very cordially enquiring how my intellectual property would be used, the responses I received instantly told me that I was not going to get anywhere with my documentary and film writing, however well-received my concepts were or whatever actual experience I had regarding the subject matter of the film, as they were all very much along the lines of: *we love this, but we want to give it to Celebrity X to present—oh, and we can't pay you for your work or give you professional credits, either, as you are unestablished.*

Or: *good idea and writing but being unknown means that audiences won't watch your work.*

That was understandable in a sense from their point of view: in them wanting to use a name for the role. But the point is that I am not sure what anyone expected me to do in that regard, as I could only offer who I am as a creative.

At the same time, I was still receiving comments urging me, due to the combination of my experiences and speaking style, to pursue something along the lines of motivational speaking, given my experiences and my overcoming them. However, at first, it felt most arrogant to me personally to even consider the idea of doing anything where one is expected to impart some kind of advice to others and so I pushed back against the idea. But it would not be my intention to provide advice in any case, rather just to contribute what was to be learned from what I had lived through and how, from that, certain relevant matters could be improved. I had been told that I had a very healthy attitude to managing adversity and I knew, somewhat instinctively perhaps, how to get through tough experiences, with, it seems, something of a strengthened mindset in some ways. I also find that encouraging bringing out the best in others can be a joy. With this in mind, I felt that perhaps there was actually something possibly helpful that I could contribute as a speaker, as had been suggested to me. I knew this would not be in any huge way, but I thought I might as well add something constructive with my experience.

However, any of this type of speaking, for me, would prove not to be the best of choices.

But that is hindsight for you.

Well, I was referred to a few speaking agencies where I was told that I could incorporate my writing, voice style and life experience. I did not want to be put into the category of a motivational or inspirational speaker, as this felt ridiculous to me, especially as I did not assume that people needed me to motivate them (I have observed that there are many people, from all areas of society, who actually do not lack motivation but it is often something related to circumstance, in any part of life, that is essentially the issue for them) plus I most certainly did not feel 'inspirational' at all. But I didn't really fit into any category of that kind of professional speaking. Most of the agencies were very nice to me, with one responding eagerly that they found me really interesting and telling me that they loved the style and content of my speaking and writing. However, they all ultimately decided that, again, my not being a name and with no media profile was too much of an issue to risk taking me on, as people simply would not know who I was.

This was fine though, and I could totally accept this view.

One person however, sent me a most curt reply stating that those from reality TV were of particular interest and that therefore what I had to say would not matter. That is no big deal, of course, but I had to wonder logically how my—and maybe others'—particular life experiences and potential contributions to the relevant fields were oh-so-meaningless in contrast to the apparently profound musings associated with appearing on a reality show.

A small part of my would-be work as a speaker was meant to be geared towards improving knowledge of female health in regard to cervical cancer. Young women had repeatedly asked me to speak about this and considering I did not want any other female to go through what I had been forced to, I felt obliged to at least use my experience to improve matters a little.

Besides which, some of the doctors had told me that I was experienced enough and knew enough about such matters, to be able to educate on such things: 'Well, you're an expert on this', said one of them, leaving me dumfounded. Though that is a most generous compliment, I do not think that I am an expert of course. It is the case though, that I can helpfully solidly contribute to this subject, even if only in some small way, and it seemed such a shame for that to go to waste.

However, it became apparent that those who would be selected to help with this subject were chosen solely on the basis of their public profile)—and, as I did not have that status, it was a no-go, regardless of whatever suitable knowledge or experience I might possess and therefore, my offers of help were always turned away.

But I recognised that I was never going to be accepted to contribute to this due to my lack of being known. One person of certain echelons of social status informed me that helping with certain causes in this way, especially speaking about them, was only for a select few of my industry and those within particular social circles, and that I would not be able to add my experience in this context. I tried not to take their attitude to heart, so I learned to get over it, but the comments made me afraid to further offer my help, despite others urging me to use my experience to make perhaps some difference.

Although travel could now be difficult for me with my health problems, I so desired to get back to seeing other countries as I had set off to do before becoming ill, when I had visited wonderful Australia with Ethan. As I wandered, in my search for the peace and rebuilding of my life that eluded me, I visited different places. I considered relocating to a couple of them, as though my homeland is lovely, as are many of the British people too, some natural environments are beneficial for my physical health. However, the practical issues surrounding work and health matters meant that this would be either impossible or unsafe. During that time, I encountered some very decent people, who kindly made time for me.

Over time, the sort of motivational-style speaking was suggested to me again and some who got to know me a little, mentioned that the style and content of my speaking might be appreciated in Monaco, as speakers of different categories work there.

But a wave of self-doubt crashed over me: it felt like a big leap from being a possible speaker in the UK, to being one in Monaco with no working up to that in between, and I was also not sure what I could offer to audiences in Monaco in terms of the content of my speaking. Though I had some knowledge and life experience in certain things, so did those in that type of an audience in other areas—and they had achieved some great things with it. But having been told that my life experiences and the views resulting from them might have relevance to some of the humanitarian issues that some support, I supposed that there was at least some relevance to it.

But a nagging doubt remained that this was perhaps not the right way forward for making anything good of what had happened to me. I did not realise that I was trying to make sense of what I had lived through by channelling the experiences into something that could do some good, except, at the time being distracted by trauma and unable to rebuild my life, this was the wrong way to go about it.

However, I was advised to find the courage to just try it out and see. So, I reluctantly gave it a go.

Some in Monaco were friendly to me, though I never got to know anyone there properly. I was suffering badly from the effects of the cancer treatment and what I had lived through, though I made every effort not to show it. I could not tell any of those who I briefly met there about my unusual life; only tiny excerpts of it when asked, such as having had cancer, or that I was a writer but trying to fully develop my creativity in other parts of the arts also, as I found it impossible to talk about myself or my life due to the bizarreness of it in that moment. My particular life experiences are not something that one can just blurt out in a normal, light-conversational situation—especially not to strangers. It would have been odd to do so. I had not anticipated this at all; I had only prepared myself for the actual talk that I might give.

There are appropriate situations in which to discuss such things —indeed, in the setting of a professional talk, that is probably one of the most ideal places—but to get onto such dark subjects to happy people chatting casually about business and enjoying the sunshine while sitting by the glistening shores of the Cote d'Azur on a beautiful summer day, is definitely not one of them.

I did not want to depress them with that, and I hugely struggled with how to translate my experiences in a business environment. As such, I became at a loss to know what to say in this instance.

My difficulties in explaining my experiences and the helpful issues that I could contribute these to by way of the professional speaking, were further impeded by being in pain from walking frequently in the heat, which had aggravated the lymphoedema, and my discomfort was visible, though thankfully nobody that I met realised how much pain I was in, as I managed to conceal it successfully.

Consequently, the combination of these aspects meant that I got no further with the motivational speaking.

Dejected, I sought solace in the delightful Princess Grace rose garden, reflective in its namesake's elegance and beauty. It was a hot day, and I sat in an almost meditative state there amongst the flowers in their splendid bloom—nature being my comforter, as always— trying to manage the pain and feeling foolish; *what on Earth was I thinking?* I ruminated. I had known that something along the lines of motivational speaking was not what I really wanted to do but had thought that I should at least give it a chance when it was suggested to me as being suitable for utilizing my life experience for. Now however, it seemed very much so like the wrong decision—and as far as I was concerned, it was one of my own making—to have even attempted to take this route and perhaps especially not in Monaco, where its audiences are accustomed to very dynamic speakers and highly achieving businesspeople, of which I was neither.

Back in the UK, I decided that it was obvious that professional speaking of that type was not for me. In Monaco I had struggled to know how to go about achieving anything as a speaker, while elsewhere I had repeatedly been told that though the content of my speaking was considered to be very appealing, it would not matter how well my words were received however, as I could never be a professional speaker unless I was a name or in the media, and so I simply left it at that. I came to realise that actually my first instinct about it was correct and that it was never for me personally: I am far better suited to putting anything that might be received as uplifting or helpful, into my creative works.

But the experience taught me that, though you will not think it at the time, such experiences can often lead you to where you *should* be in life.

For some time now, I had been riding my bike to the treatment appointments for the after-effects of the cancer, and one day after leaving one of these, I felt an urge to look at the buildings in which my life had partly been ruined. I knew that the buildings had been abandoned a few years previously and were derelict now, and I had not seen them since my diagnosis many years earlier. I felt strangely drawn to them. I do not know what I hoped to get out of seeing them, though I knew it felt important to me. Hence, I took a detour through the large medical complexes and first, headed to the building where I had been almost forced into inappropriate care for the symptoms of my cancer being classed as 'psychosomatic'. The large, gloomy building was being demolished.

As I sat on my bike, staring at the building with its missing, torn-down side wall, suddenly, an extremely uncharacteristic feeling began to well up inside of me, something I had never really felt before, in the form of indignation. I stared at the building, trying to make sense of my feelings: some kind of vague embarrassing chagrin, mixed with the strangeness of my experiences and intense violation.

You know, this is not spoken about, but I feel that some, me included, who have survived extraordinary things that are, through no fault of their own, irregular and have an element of the bizarre to them, often find that this is one of the hardest things about the ordeal to process: the strangeness; the weird element of the experience. In my case, I felt deeply embarrassed over the weirdness of the ordeals that I had been subjected to. Here, looking at one of the places where I had been degraded during the misdiagnosis, this abashment enveloped me.

Afterwards, I cycled through the complex to the building that bothered me the most: an old laboratory building that had been abandoned—peculiarly, just after my cancer diagnosis—and that had been involved in my cervical screening testing. It was quiet here and nobody was around. Earmarked for demolition, a cordon had been placed around the abandoned, run-down building. The slight ray of daylight shining through one of the building's broken windows revealed that there was still discarded medical equipment remaining. I had a strong urge to enter the building and look around it; to see if there was any evidence remaining of what had been going on in there. I knew it would be wrong to do so, however, and so I simply stared at it, trying to make sense of what had happened and the intense feelings that I was now trying to process.

What did they do to me in there? I found myself wondering.

I pictured the building in full working use and what the people working there might have been doing in their work and how they had, allegedly, not adhered to the regulations of their profession.

But then I saw the place for exactly what it was. *It is just a building,* I thought, *that is all. An abandoned building that no longer holds any capacity to cause any harm to anyone.*

In a strange kind of way, I guess I was experiencing what we might call closure (though does this ever fully exist?): seeing the buildings, especially the laboratory, as unnerving as it was for me, brought my true feelings about not being believed for so many years about my cancer symptoms to the fore. It settled something for me, though I never knew quite what or how.

But what I did now understand was that in order to maintain a healthy mindset, I had to let go of my intense feelings of indignation, shame, and violation there and then; to leave them there, with these places, in the past.

15
Running Down the Wrong Road

WHILST MY REVISITING THE PLACES that had played such a crucial role in the catastrophic route of my life had settled some feelings for me, in other ways, it had brought up some very uneasy emotions, too, a particularly overwhelming one of which being guilt—an intense guilt that I had failed the others who had been affected by misread testing—and I felt that it was an issue that some needed to be informed of, for the sake of the health, or, as it is no exaggeration to say, the lives, of others. I began thinking that, in retrospect, perhaps I should have agreed to some of the legal advice about this aspect of what had happened: that is, the press aspect, and how it might have helped others.

There is no way that I would agree to be a part of a media spotlight myself however, because besides my never feeling a need to be at the forefront of anything, I carried intense embarrassment about what had happened to me.

But now it occurred to me that maybe what I could do instead was find a trustworthy and sensible journalistic advocate of sorts who might be appropriate to further the help that I had tried to provide.

Hence, this is what my conscience, against my better judgement, led me to do. Eventually, I gave in to my guilt for not doing enough about the situation with the other possible cervical screening cases. The matter was troubling me, prompting me to try and amend a little of what I had been advised to do regarding the possibility of issues with misdiagnosis cases but was terrified of; speak to the press. But this would only be so to contribute a few words on the matter, preferably in writing, and with the intention of trying to help with the wider cause of implementing real change to protect others' health and lives regarding this issue, by privately raising the concerns surrounding it.

However, upon vaguely enquiring into this a few times, though one journalist was nice to me, their colleague then sent me a scornful response telling me that they had important people who had appeared in the media to work with and that having no public profile whatsoever, I was considered very unimportant indeed. That was fair enough; but they had not seemed to realise that the important element of this had nothing to do with whoever I was but was in fact the rather concerning and urgent matter of the cervical screening issues.

Eventually, I found what I thought to be an appropriate person who appeared to be interested—though the person came across as somewhat brash and pushy. Upon my explanation of the misdiagnosis and other possible cases (though mine was deemed somewhat distinct in terms of my having a longer misdiagnosis, the unnecessary psychological-analyses and also due to some of the effects of the cancer treatment), they demanded to see information in order to decide if I was worth taking seriously.

Overlooking their abruptness, I sent them some relevant information at their request, having been assured that it would be entirely strictly confidential—and with this, Pushy Person, though they now realised that I was genuine, then went on to ask me for more and more sensitive and private details.

Feeling unsure about that, I told them that I needed to take some time to think about the way forward with this. I then spent three months trying to decide what to do in my turmoil; I was fighting feelings of fear over speaking to the media so that I could do the right thing by societal expectations. This ultimately cancelled out my own wellbeing, even when doing something that I did not feel at all comfortable with—and so I contacted Pushy Person to tell them of my decision to say a little of something to maybe prompt a change in matters, in order to perhaps help to save lives.

The extraordinary conversation that ensued would leave me regretting having ever decided to reluctantly take this route in regard to my experiences with the cervical screening issues.

The requests for information became more and more personal and seemed to point towards doing a newspaper feature revealing my innermost trauma and private life. This was not at all what I had contacted them for, and I declined to do it. 'This is about very serious and worrying issues that have endangered lives,' I said gently.

But Pushy Person responded nonchalantly, 'So what? Not your story.'

I responded by politely explaining that as I was the most severely affected survivor, and who had the lengthiest misdiagnosis, as well as the person who had helped uncover the possibility of more misread testing cases, therefore the subject could not be any more relevant to me indeed, though however, I wanted those details to be kept private, as I didn't want to be seen as some kind of victim.

But it did not matter anyway as they said they were not interested in that.

Instead, I listened to Pushy Person telling me how they thought an editor would want an article of this nature to look, going completely off-course from the purposes that I had intended with the subject.

Pushy Person wanted pictures of Ethan and I for use in an article. I would not provide them, I said, and I do not want to discuss my life in this manner. I politely explained that Ethan wished to maintain his privacy and does not appear in the media. *They will, of course, understand that*, I thought. *All of the press understands that in these such situations, don't they?*

Astonishingly, though, Pushy Person replied, 'I don't buy that. These ex-military blokes who say that they don't want to be in the media… It's rubbish. No one will even be interested in looking at him. No one would notice him in the picture.'

Stunned at the ignorance of that comment but puzzled at the contradiction, I logically asked, 'But if no one is interested in looking at him, then why do you need his picture?'

Pushy Person was beginning to get annoyed. 'Because people will want to see pictures of your life', they snapped.

'But I don't feel a need to show pictures of my life,' I responded.

'Well, the editor will want to print them,' they said. Their reaction to my refusal to play ball in being part of a tacky media article was to try and push the matter further, 'They will also want to know about your sex life. They will want you to describe how the cancer treatment has affected your sex life.'

I wondered where on Earth that topic had come from. *I have never told them or anyone else anything whatsoever relating to that subject, so why do they just assume that they know what had affected me and how? Do they ever consider that things might not be like they imagine at all?* I thought.

(My sensuality, in actual fact, had been unaffected, but being expected to explain that publicly felt degrading).

Given that the only subject that I was meant to be discussing was that of the concerning cervical screening issues, I was baffled as to why all of these other things were now popping up in the form of questions and expectations.

Now way out of my depth, I could only reply with, 'I'm sorry, but I will not talk about any personal things in the media. Can you please tell the editor that I do not want to discuss such personal details about myself?'

Pushy Person, annoyed at my response, exclaimed, 'These are *editors* that you are talking about; you show them some respect!'

To this, I was unsure what possibly to say, but tried to be diplomatic, 'It has taken me a lot of holding my nerve together to be able to find it in me to come to those like you regarding the cervical screening cases. That was what I felt should be discussed, not for me to talk about my personal life in the media.'

Declining to be photographed in the press or discuss personal things led to Pushy Person continuing loudly, 'I am telling you now, I am not putting up with this.'

I did not know in that moment what to say or how to handle this situation. I suddenly realised that this had been a serious error of judgement on my part, and that I should have stuck with my original strong, instinctive feeling that this route of trying to bring about change and improvement for the screening cases was not right for me.

But I managed to say, 'I brought to you a very serious situation whereby some women have died of cancer or been affected by it, when it potentially could have been prevented. Surely that is more important to people than talking about my private life?'

'No, it isn't,' said Pushy Person. 'People want to read about personal details. They want to know about people's sex lives. That's why people like features on celebrity affairs.'

I thought that to be insulting to the majority of newspaper readers, who I expected were not so small-minded that all they found scintillating in media articles was, essentially, trash.

Regardless, Pushy Person continued, 'Look, no one will be interested in you because you're reluctant to be in the media, you don't want anything to do with reality TV, you won't share personal details about yourself on social media, and you have absolutely no controversy in your life. *You* are the one with the problem. There is nothing we can work with other than if you tell us about your sex life. The readers will want to know about that. People want to read about what affects relationships. That's why things like kiss-and-tell stories sell newspapers.'

'I don't understand,' I responded, confused, 'the information that I came to you with is nothing at all to do with any of that kind of thing. Certainly, neither am I. But in any case, readers frequently state how they are sick of trash in the media. Like them, I think it is not what many of us want to read about. I think that profound journalism is extremely important, but this is something different; all this other stuff is just tacky. It's not anything I personally want to be a part of. This is not what I contacted you for; it was meant to be about the cervical screening cases. But as you have brought the subject up, I agree with some others: I would also prefer to see more of the people featured in the media who have standards and values instead of those doing kiss-and-tell stories and trashy nonsense.'

Pushy Person then exploded with rage at my words. '*Standards and values*? That is *absolutely* disgusting!'

In my life so far, my experiences at the hands of others who demanded my subservience had conditioned me to think their voice to be more important than mine. Hence, I just continued to listen to them rant. Realising the situation that I had gotten myself into with inadvertently enraging a person within the media, I felt overwhelmed about this.

It was the middle of winter and a gloomy, overcast day. As I knelt to the floor in the kitchen, the room was dark with rain pattering down the windows, and this somehow reflected the way that I felt in that moment. Pushy Person continued loudly ranting, 'Standards and values! *All* of the people I work with have standards and values!'

In that moment, a couple of media articles popped into my mind that completely contradicted that statement, leaving me slightly in confusion. However, that was none of my business and so I said nothing about those. Besides which, I now felt fear at how this person might choose to use their power over me if I said anything to annoy them further, given how they wanted to write the type of article that would further add to the embarrassment that I felt over my experiences.

Knowing that I had to stand up for my principles, I replied very softly but diplomatically, 'Well, it's a subject that I rarely mention. But the reason I did so in this particular instance was because it is appropriate, as I am one of the *many* people—all manner of people—who are conscious of their own personal values and know what they won't do or condone, if being persuaded to—and I won't condone trashy articles or take part in that world. That was specifically what I was referring to in regard to standards and values.'

How, I wondered, had I contacted this person with such serious information and been reduced to this demeaning conversation, in which they had, for some reason, strayed into an entirely different topic of which was nothing at all to do with me or what I had contacted them about? My refusal to go along with tacky media articles had somehow led to my having to justify the apparently preposterous notion of why I, like a great many other people the world over, think values and some kind of standards and principles to have importance.

When questioned further, I managed to say, 'No matter how much someone humiliates me for them, my principles and values are at the very core of who I am. I am sorry, but that is my stance on these matters. I do not ever get involved with debates or tell others what to do, but if I am being told that I should abandon my principles to go along with the idea that tacky or manipulative stories are good, then I cannot do that.'

Pushy Person then loudly and mockingly exclaimed, '*Your* principles! *Your* values! Who cares about *your* principles and values? Who would want to know *anything* about what *you* think or what *you* have to say?'

I could barely form a reply, at the unnerving thought of what I had gotten myself into with this person within the media but downheartedly answered. 'Well, I absolutely do not expect that people *do* want to know about them or to hear from me, and I don't ever speak about such things usually, but then I have no desire whatsoever to tell anyone what to do. I only mentioned such things to you because it was relevant. However, separately in my writing, I have received kind comments from people saying that they like my words, including from professionals within the arts and film.'

Pushy Person then exclaimed with ridicule, '*You've* been told that? An unknown like *you*?!'

As the effects of my life experiences and the cancer treatment sometimes intensify when under stress, I now felt unwell, but humiliatingly answered that yes, this was in fact the case.

They now responded in a completely normal tone, 'All that is, is that you have allowed yourself to be *flattered*. Let me give you some advice: people won't read your writing and the production companies will not use it even if it's really good because you are not famous; they're just flattering you. Your life experience and even what you are good at, means nothing because you are unknown. You have *allowed* yourself to be *flattered*. It's easily done. I'm telling you the truth here.'

'Well,' I politely replied, 'it seemed to be most genuine. I am acutely aware of the difference.'

Pushy Person's voice changed to a quiet and mocking tone, as they stated randomly, 'Are you *special*? Is Rebecka *special*?' They then changed tone of voice again and angrily continued, 'Who would want to know about *you*? Who would want to hear *you* speak or hear *your* opinion? Who are *you* to think that anyone will want to read your writing or watch your documentaries? I will tell you who you are, Rebecka: *you're nobody.*'

Sensing that I had not spoken in some time, Pushy Person paused and calmed their voice. In a completely composed manner, they said, 'You've gone silent just because you're shocked. Being spoken to like this is a shock to you because nobody would ever have told you anything like this before; that you are not special or that anything that you have to say is important.' (my silence was actually a dignified one).

Informing them of the facts being to the absolute contrary would be pointless; they simply would not listen. So, I instead replied solemnly, 'I really do not think myself to be special in any way at all. I never have done. I do not expect that anyone would be interested in my views, but then it is not my opinion that I wanted to share; I keep my opinions to myself, generally. It was just some knowledge that I felt obligated to share regarding extremely serious issues related to female health that could have been very helpful to many others' wellbeing and possibly save lives.'

Pushy Person continued now in a normal, unraised and calm tone, 'Well, I think you need to be told. I'm trying to give you advice here. I'm not being horrible to you—I think you're really sweet—but I am not afraid to tell anyone about themselves. I've been offered many roles to give my opinions, and I don't take the offers up, but I'm not afraid to tell anyone what I think of them, and I'm not afraid to tell *you*; you are *nobody*, Rebecka, yeah? No one will ever have told you that you are nothing.'

If only they knew...

Although this bizarre and degrading phone conversation adversely affected my sense of self for some time, I hold no ill feeling towards the person and do not wish this experience to detract from any of the nice people in the media. But, having been shy of this arena before, I was now rendered acutely so.

Oddly, this experience helped to settle my constant feeling of being torn between a troubled social conscience regarding the cervical screening issues and other possible cases and then my fear of partaking in the media regarding that (therefore perhaps not doing the right thing by others in the process), along with my reservedness and the effects of the way that I was extensively mistreated in the misdiagnosis, I decided that my true feelings were that I never wanted to talk about it again: I had done all that I could manage in terms of trying to help with this issue in order to protect others and with nothing more that I could do about it, doing so was badly damaging my wellbeing.

The feeling of some kind of closure that I had previously obtained by visiting the abandoned medical buildings was now strengthened by the realisation that it was harming my health to pursue this matter further.

Perhaps if someone had taken notice of the issues that my experiences had raised and the changes that I was trying to help implement, then things could have been improved. But my lack of media profile or connections deemed me unworthy of ever being taken seriously in this regard.

I could not go on like this any longer. The knowledge of this issue was a huge responsibility to bear, and I was prevented at every turn from doing anything helpful with it. I had never invited my involvement in this into my life but had truly done all that I could, in my circumstances, to help (at least ensuring as much as possible that what had happened to me couldn't happen to anyone else in future), though I was restricted with what I could achieve with this. This situation was draining me and damaging my health. Ethan told me, 'You've done your bit and that's enough'. This made sense, though at the time I felt troubled by not doing more to help. But feeling completely overwhelmed by this situation and knowing that this was not at all how I wanted to live my life, I realised that in order to remain a well-balanced person, I should now let it go and leave it all here.

This decision would prove in time to be most conducive to my wellbeing and, with nothing left of myself to give, I had made the right choice in that regard by leaving the whole matter of the cervical screening fiasco behind and not discussing it anymore.

(The cervical screening would later become much improved, and, in spite of my developing cervical cancer, the testing is indeed absolutely crucial for saving many lives and should always be undertaken).

Shortly prior to the embarrassing phone conversation, some friendly ladies involved in the world of famous comedy performers had welcomed me into their professional world as a potential writer. Whilst the comedy ladies knew hardly anything about my experiences (I would never tell anyone the extent of that), they were understanding about the very little that they did know of. They appreciated that my writing was multidimensional and that though I could write earnestly for profound subjects, my style could also separately be humorous in execution—a combination that is not at all unusual among writers of TV or film production.

There is often never as much humour as in absurdity, I feel—and I have observed plenty of that throughout my life.

I can certainly laugh at myself too.

To cry with laughter is wonderful and I believe that laughter should be entirely pure and never just offered for the sake of it, and definitively never false.

Enforced joviality is, I believe, the realm of the insane.

Good humour, to me, just like good music, often unites people in the best of ways.

Well, the comedy ladies invited me to submit some of my writing, as they liked a couple of my ideas, and I was very grateful of this. I was not hired to write anything at this stage, but I was permitted to submit my concepts for perusal.

I was beginning work on adapting some of my concepts possibly for screen around the time that the demeaning conversation with Pushy Person occurred, after which I felt that I could never again face writing anything to be submitted for film or TV, considering what the person had told me in that conversation about how people were only flattering me about my work. I now suddenly felt as though I was fooling myself into thinking that I could ever possibly have my work brought to the screen.

Pushy Person's voice and opinion spoke to me louder than that of the friendly professional comedy ladies: that is the wrong way round, as I would later learn, but I could not help it at the time as I now just suddenly had an overwhelming feeling of not being good enough for this professional world of supreme talent. I never told anyone in the business how I was feeling: it was my way to always keep my struggles to myself as I did not want to bother anyone with them. I was now rendered extremely reluctant to submit any of my writing ever again.

While in the process of trying to find what to do with the possible artistry that I was encouraged to use, I also sought other ways that I could utilize a combination of my creativity and life experience. I was referred to the editor of a stylish magazine, which also included articles concerning serious matters, to discuss working on an engaging piece or feature for them. However, as usual, having no public profile and being an unknown meant that the magazine's editorial team were not interested.

With my health problems, as a result of the cancer, finally beginning to become under control, I wanted to return to some of the things that I had done previously. A photographer said that they would like to photograph me for a fashion and arts magazine. I had not been expecting this and felt very touched by this gesture. I replied with much gratitude, having been turned away from anything connected to style or photography since having the cancer. For the purposes of the photoshoot, I explained very briefly, so as not to overwhelm them with information, a little mention of the lymphoedema, as I thought that given the nature of their associate's charity work for issues surrounding cancer, they would be understanding about it. However, I received a very curt reply from them stating that they were fully booked for the rest of the year and would probably never be able to work with me. The mere mention of a miniscule part of my experiences and illness had entirely put the photographer off working with me, when if they had met me, they would have seen that unless I was experiencing a particularly bad day with the illness, there was no actual indicator of the lymphoedema at all to someone who is not a medical professional, and that it would not cause any issues for working with me.

Shame enveloped me in relation to this; I was not sure what people were expecting to see in regards to the lymphoedema, the cancer treatment, and the extensive irregular and unpleasant life experiences when they met me, but it nearly always comes as a huge surprise to them when they see that there is no outward sign at all of what I have endured: I look very healthy and have mostly maintained the gait and posture that I obtained through the professional disciplines that I have trained in. Thanks to keeping the lymphoedema in check, in my particular case, with regular lymphatic drainage massage and being as active as I possibly can, with ballet and cycling being the most effective forms of managing the illness for me personally (I cannot speak for others who have lymphoedema as each individual case should be advised by a medical professional, but as exercise is crucial to keeping the illness under control, in my own personal case I have found that the lymphoedema responds as optimally as possible to resistance training in addition to lymphatic drainage).

However, I came to realise that most people had not heard of lymphoedema and consequently, many of those who I had to mention it to, would then, not believing that it is an illness, simply because they had never heard of it, Google it, leading to their reading of articles showing the extreme end of the illness (which I do not have, but which very sadly, affects some). This would then lead them to assume this would be representative of me, which is very much not the case. Since intensive treatment at the specialist lymphoedema hospital overseas, the lymphoedema had actually become undetectable most of the time to anyone who did not know how to look for it (though I would always have some slight problem with swelling on my lower abdomen, directly where I had the surgery and so many lymph nodes removed) and I even receive compliments on how nice my legs apparently look, with people being completely unaware that I have lymphoedema. I wear compression when exercising or taking a flight, but otherwise people cannot even tell that I suffer from the illness. Though it causes me pain on a daily basis, irrespective of how in check it might be, my physique was now returning back to what it had been before. I also have a normal walk.

My illness is not a label for me to wear but is in fact, a mere embuggerance. It is the least interesting thing about me. I feel self-conscious of my health problems (which are physical and entirely stem from the effects of the cancer), but also, crucially, they are not the focal point of who I am, so I don't speak about them or mention them whenever I can avoid doing so. Instead, this is how I deal with them: I carry-on as I would otherwise have done as much as possible, with what I want to do with my life and focus on expression of some kind of beauty and passion in what I can create.

People talk to me all the time while being completely oblivious to what I have lived through (and that is completely fine by me).

As for the swelling post-cancer treatment, learning what works for me personally in how to control it, I would go on to eventually manage it successfully and to wear pretty shoes, shorts and dresses with abandon.

So, it seemed perhaps foolish for others who had not met me to build an image in their mind of what they expected me to be given what I have survived, without even entertaining the idea that I am actually nothing like that at all.

The paradox in regard to this that I observed, however, was that we sometimes see, especially on social media and in the media in general, some who seem to thrive on the attention drawn from creating dramatic situations through their own behaviour again and again, for goodness knows what reason. I take no interest in the goings-on of such histrionics generally, but the point is that I could not help but be puzzled at this one simple repeated observation: bad or abnormal behaviour in this regard is now seen as being acceptable—even enabled or normalized in some cases—whilst the experiences that have happened to myself that I had not invited and had no control over would often prompt some element of shame.

It was also confusing and difficult to understand how some whom seemed to be so publicly supportive of cancer causes, would abruptly no longer speak to me once they learned of my cancer and a tiny part of the experiences surrounding it.

I was confused by their contradictory behaviour at first and could not understand it but as I would notice at times in life—and there would be more of them—while there are people who do amazing humanitarian and philanthropic things to help others (and all love to them, they are wonderful people), it is unfortunate that there are others for whom being *seen* to be humanitarian and charitable can serve them very well.

However, I tried not to take it to heart.

While navigating being on the receiving end of such attitudes, I decided to focus on developing myself as a creative, even if I was shunned by some due to the circumstances of my life.

However, being repeatedly told that my abilities met the necessary professional standards but that my life and circumstances as an unknown with no connections deemed me unable to get anywhere with them, meant that my eternal predicament remained.

Timing, too, had consistently been a factor. Both of these aspects seemed to play an important role in getting anywhere within the professional fields of the arts and entertainment that I had been ushered into for so long.

These things had held me back so much for years, when I had tried to achieve something in my earlier life—and then just as I was overcoming them and proper interest in working with me was beginning to be shown, I received the cancer diagnosis. Now, I was back to square one, with the added elements of what I had since survived.

Some say that we make our own luck in life. I agree with that — up to a point. I think that true success is a formula: the vast majority of which being personal effort, responsibility, self-discipline, and of course, the obviously required skill or talent. However, the formula also requires an added tiny pinch of that perhaps not-so-mysterious ingredient made up of opportunity that makes the whole recipe come together.

My angst at this seemingly never-ending cycle grew. I simply needed the opportunity to be able to do something good with my creative work.

So, when one day Ethan said, 'You know all the compliments that you receive on your voice? Well, why don't you get into the studio and start recording? You could work easily around your health problems doing that', I felt that this would perhaps be a far more sensible choice for me, given my predicament.

Because of the very lengthy misdiagnosis, I had barely had the opportunity to do anything as a performer, including in voiceover, and on the few occasions I had been asked to record in the past, it had come naturally to me, and I had been incredibly comfortable with working in the studio. However, there was one problem: that was, my voice being affected by my experiences in that it would sometimes, in certain situations, fade, effectively, 'losing' my voice, having been shouted down and told to shut up for such a long time by those who felt it was their place to do so, whenever I tried to speak up for myself. Therefore, I was concerned that my professional speaking voice would never return to normal.

However, I was delighted to find that in speaking professionally, the reverse of this happened: when recording again, I felt very comfortable indeed. There was no threat to me whatsoever here in the recording studio: no belittling of who I was or what I had lived through. Hence, my voice was perfectly fine and now permanently always would be. I could just be completely free with letting my voice do its stuff, finding that it was still clear and I received great feedback on the recording from some of the industry professionals, who classed my voice style as 'eloquent and soothing' and confirmed that it's warmth and smoothness was still present. 'It's great, Beck. Pretty cool. You will have no problem getting back with an agency for representation in the arts.' And as it would turn out, they were right; I was accepted onto the books of one in London and later one overseas also. I was a complete unknown in a world of some of the most supreme talent of the performing arts and though I was nothing at all among them, it was a privilege to be accepted by them.

My literacy skills could also be utilised for complex scripts or those with an extensive vocabulary. However, though I was comfortable in my abilities, I certainly did not think myself to be of the wonderous talent of the greats of voiceover.

The use of my particular voice style is only one of the aspects of my being a creative, but it was a start.

This was what I should have been doing all along. Finally, I was on the right path. That was thanks to Ethan's suggestion.

'Your voice would be perfect for fantasy film,' I was told by a professional in voiceover, 'but unfortunately you will never be able to use it in that way because only famous actors are chosen for that.' They did, however, tell me that my lack of fame might not hold me back from audiobook narration, where they felt that audiences would apparently be drawn to the soft and relaxing tone of my voice.

Around this time, further interest was also taken in my writing on a very small scale. But I was told once again that I would never get any further with publishing any of my writing for book or film production because, in effect, I was unconnected to anyone or anything seemingly significant.

Someone in the arts who had complimented my voice and writing told me, while well-intentioned, 'It doesn't matter how good you look, if you have a lovely voice, how people love your words, how much life experience you have, you will never get any further with your creative work because you are unknown. You are not connected to anyone, and you are not on TV.' But I could do nothing about being unknown or my lack of connections and I never had any desire to be on TV.

As usual, I only wanted to focus on the possible artistry of what I had been selected to do professionally and therefore could see no way of overcoming the view of why already being a public persona or having connections was considered to be the defining factor to some when it comes to offering what one may have as a creative.

I wondered though if I was yet again going to be held back by circumstance—but no matter: I was going to make the best of my situation.

In my quest to rebuild my life, I had taken the wrong path several times in trying to find my way again.

But now I knew that what I was very much cut out for, as I was professionally advised in my early life, was translating life, emotions, and characters into word form, either in a written or spoken performance capacity, producing that of (hopefully) beauty, connection, humour, or comfort in the process.

For years, due to my unfortunate start in life, and then because of the consequences of the misdiagnosis, cancer treatment, and rehabilitation, I had been prevented from at all progressing properly as a creative professional.

But now, with great effort and never-ending perseverance, I had finally found some direction—a starting point—to fit in professionally and begin the process of rebuilding my life.

Despite all the odds, and, after all the effort, humiliation, hardship and pain, I had succeeded in adapting to the experiences that had been forced upon me and overcoming the many obstacles that I had faced, now with a renewed sense of hope for making something good of my life.

Ultimately, I found a little of my place in the world—right where it had been from my early years: within the creative world; a place where I could at last begin to flourish.

16
Crushed

HAVING BEEN REPEATEDLY URGED TO use the combination of my experiences and manner of speaking and writing to help in a sort of advocational way with certain issues that my life experiences had relevance to, I felt that perhaps that might make some sense.

However, as it had been with the public speaking, I felt greatly uncomfortable putting myself forward for this. To me, it felt arrogant doing so. But I did not want others to go through what I had experienced or witnessed. So, when I was made aware of, through the social media that I had for my work as a creative, a few charities that I felt I had some measure of relevance to and perhaps something of a wealth of experience for some, I was willing to help by offering to write a few articles for them or to contribute my experience and understanding to a concept to further their work, but they always, though in a polite manner, turned me away due to my complete lack of being known and not being a high profile person.

This was fair enough.

Certainly, I do not have all the answers, nor am I a crusader or activist for such matters. I also wanted to help as privately as possible, not be at the forefront or involved in the media side of things. I just thought it sensible to utilize my life experience of the subjects, to help implement additional progress being made. I had noticed that because the wider picture is often left unseen, things never really improve for some, and they are forgotten about, and I could also help with improving educated understanding of matters.

In these respects, perhaps there might be something of value that I could add.

This is what I offered, with politeness and without fuss, to contribute and to privately offer a bit of dignified constructive input for, in the hopes that it would prompt an improvement in the quality of life for those who are very much so in need of that or to help implement something effectual.

However, this was clearly not something that I would be accepted to do; regardless of my experience, being unknown and with no public profile or connections meant that I was always turned down from contributing in this way.

Paradoxically, after being told that I was not important enough to do so, some made a point of letting me know that I was *not* helping enough with charitable issues, especially compared to them. In a couple of instances in this regard, it was strange to be told by some who did not have my relevant life experiences of certain matters— but considered themselves to be expert on the issues connected to them—who the hell did I think I was offering my help, especially given that, as they told me, they saw me as being nothing. I did not respond or explain my relevance to the issues and was instead perfectly content to let them bask in the spotlight and admiration that they craved. I had happily never needed that.

In actual fact, they did not know that the docufilm concepts and written pieces that I had devised to hopefully help further understanding for the subjects, though accepted as very appealing ideas, had all been rejected on the basis of my being unknown. Neither did they know that it had been recommended professionally on occasion, that I publish writing about the subjects to bring about a greater comprehension of them. I was never going to tell them about this, because anything I might do to contribute, I like to do privately and quietly.

There are only so many times that a person can offer a bit of constructive help, based on their life experience, because ultimately you get the message; it was made perfectly clear that I was not considered to be valuable enough to help due to my having no media profile. That was absolutely fine, and I understood.

But I had tried my best to utilize my experiences to add

something of value that others could benefit from, and as an individual and unknown, I really could do no more than that.

Enthused to learn on social media of what I thought to be some possible help for Ethan through appropriate channels after I was contacted by some connected to them (though these were legitimate, that does not mean that someone will not misuse the position that they have been afforded), it was, in fact, the first time I had ever felt able to confide in anyone that I had struggled for so long in my attempts to help him with his difficulties which included practical matters. Indeed, I had rarely felt able to ask anyone for help for anything at all during my life.

They offered to help and seemed very friendly initially, so I hoped that Ethan would finally receive a bit of assistance. They increasingly asked me personal questions that were nothing to do with what I had enquired about, but I explained that I did not discuss my life and personal details on social media. It was insisted, however, with great encouragement, that I could trust them if I told them all about myself and was assured that anything I privately shared with them would be entirely confidential, though I declined to entirely do so.

When they repeatedly referred to their contacts and the influence that they held, while pointing out my insignificance, I tried not to read too much into it as I am not easily offended and so I allowed for them perhaps just being a bit too over-confident or overbearing.

But then they continued in randomly putting me down and though I can cope with that, in this instance the particular disdainful manner of it, began to leave me filled with self-doubt. Their demands for me to reveal more and more about myself and my life increased. When I refused to tell them more, they told me I was crazy.

Although this had been subtle to begin with, it now became bolder, with them getting others to join in their behaviour, on some occasions under, though I did not know it at the time, the false pretence of befriending me in order to find out more about me and by encouraging them to put me down, with the seeming intention of enjoying the possibility of any attention that this might bring them.

I thought it would be petulant to do anything about it; thinking that surely by doing so, I would be joining the fatuous behaviour of this new school playground of the constantly overbearing, besides which people are of course perfectly entitled to their freedom of expression, so I just tried to put up with this behaviour as best as I could.

But though I pleaded with them to stop this, explaining that I was trying to rebuild my life after what I had lived through, they just laughed this off and because of their dominance with their perceived status and them saying that they could help me, I continued to put up with their behaviour.

Though I was only on social media in the first place as I had been requested to be for my evolving creative work for those who wished to follow that, it had been outrightly decided by one person in particular, for some unfathomable reason, that I as a person, being a complete unknown with a new social media account, who was reserved and had a life that was very unlike theirs, was apparently too different and therefore, in their mind, could not be possible.

I could have found this comically odd if it were not for the acute viciousness of it.

Previously I had learned that, for some of a particular mindset, it is viewed as fine and celebrated, to have certain qualities or an unconventional life if one is famous—but otherwise, this is deemed completely unacceptable, especially when combined with different life experiences. Again, this is because such combinations are not the mainstream. Laura had warned me this could happen, stating that it could be 'too much for the ignorant to comprehend.' But as logical as Laura's reasoning was, it could not help me now, even though those people were in a very tiny minority, as they implied that their perceived status gave them the right to behave this way.

It later became starkly apparent what their intentions really were, as the crushingly painful realisation set in that I had allowed myself to be strung along; that some had, in fact, never genuinely cared about me or intended to help my situation at all, but simply pretended to so they could use their status to win over my trust in order to suit whatever was their intention. I realised that I had been too friendly and trusting with people, and with my past experiences of being abused in this manner, I should have known better.

I also berated myself for being too trusting in my attempt to get a little help for Ethan—whom I had never spoken about publicly and is a completely private person who has never partaken in any social media—and felt distressed that in doing so had inadvertently compromised his wellbeing. He never received the help that he had needed for so many years. I secretly often fretted that I could have done so much better in helping him to build the better quality of life that he very much deserved.

The behaviour that I was being subjected to especially by a particular person, took the form of features of the abuse that I had previously experienced in my life, including the perpetrator (others do not generally treat me this way) suggesting that I was imagining something and making it clear that there would be consequences if I did not do as they told me to (later, someone expert in being aware of this type of behaviour explained to me, "They do this so that you will give them the reaction that they want, to suit their agenda". Such behaviour would leave me in a great deal of self-doubt. Though I had mostly wised up to this in actual life, here in this unfamiliar territory of social media it had become far more difficult to spot} and here, someone felt that their apparent status gave them the right to do this.

The words of their threatening messages, in something of a diatribe, ordered me to stay away from the parts of social media that they considered to be theirs and everyone within them, and, specifically, I was ordered to stop offering my help to the charitable issues of which I had some earnest life experience and understanding of, as they told me that those issues were their domain. It was made clear in no uncertain terms that I had to obey their orders; they would use the influence that they held if I did not do as I was told, while my life experiences were derided by them through degrading words, as though I was not even a human being.

Of this, they seemed very smug.

Their behaviour, strengthened by exerting the backdrop of their authority and connections, had become an issue to being able to use the social media for what I had started it for—at request, to show my developing creative works—as attempts were made to ensure that, if others showed any kind interest in me or complimented me in any way, which many lovely people did, this was put a stop to.

Those deriving power from my angst at their efforts to ensure that I would not get any further in perhaps contributing my life experience to making a little helpful difference where needed, did not seem to realise that they had no need to humiliate me; others had already achieved that many times throughout my life and the effects of that on my sense of self had been long-lasting and had been exactly why I had struggled with the attention and public aspects of working within a professional arena that is surrounded by media. I had been told by some in the arts and media that this fear would lessen with experience of being around that side of things and indeed, this had begun to feel less daunting.

Now, I could not have felt any worse about myself.

Anyone who, like me, truly has felt what is known as 'imposter syndrome', knows that being thought to be any good at anything can come with a feeling of not being worthy of that; instead, we internalise feelings along the somewhat dramatic lines of: *you don't deserve to be here in this arena, as you don't make the grade; you're not worthy of this part; of this role; these compliments; this extension of kindness. You will be found out for fooling yourself into thinking that you were ever good enough to be here.*

We know, somewhere inside of us, that this is not true, of course, as the facts dictate that we are there, as part of something, on legitimate merit, but that realisation still does not quell such inexplicable feelings of discomfort.

For many years, I had a feeling that I should maybe not be seen or heard, especially in the public sense (this had felt at odds with being told by professionals of the arts that I apparently had something to offer as a performer and in front of the camera. My creativity being the only outlet with which to ever be able to express myself, when allowed to) and feared being in the realms of public life as a creative, which is a prospective biproduct of working in the arts that I had always struggled with. Now, in my mind, those degrading, threatening words that I had received, confirmed to me that perhaps that feeling might have been right.

I became aware that if I came close to achieving anything with my creative work or was to be perhaps kindly asked to contribute my life experience to something helpful to others in future, that would mean possibly being subject to further intimidation and this was something that on my own, I could not stand up against.

Being subjected to such experiences can be very detrimental for the state of mind indeed, even if, like me, one does not have mental illness. The insomnia that I had suffered from now worsened, as those particular threatening words played on my mind for months afterwards, culminating in a moment of distraction in rumination over them while I was riding my bike at a point where I had built up speed on it while cycling downhill and I consequently lost control of the bike and was thrown from it with force. Sustaining extensive soft tissue injuries, cuts and considerable bruising to my lymphoedema-affected areas, I was treated at the hospital's emergency department.

That was the turning point: I could not go on like this any longer. *Was I going to let this experience affect what was left of the life that I had barely ever had the chance to start living properly?*

On a more uplifting note, aside from that crushingly awful experience, all others on social media that I encountered (though of course, being completely unknown, very few people even knew of my extremely minor presence on there) were absolutely lovely in their messages and comments.

When considering certain aspects of social media, it might be imperative to bear in mind that there are actually many really good people on there, from all walks of life and from all over the world (along with many businesses and charities who possess truly good ethics), but they perhaps just get drowned out by a sea of ego and idiotic noise, which is why we often think that social media is profoundly dreadful—and, indeed, parts of it can be (I do not get involved in any of the conflict on social media as I am not confrontational or highly opinionated. Though we may not want to see it or comment on it, we are unwittingly are exposed to it any way), and it is unavoidable to notice that there is an unsettling side to some aspects of social media that hide under the impression of something with good intentions, but which perhaps have ulterior motives.

The decent people therefore sometimes go largely unnoticed

because of this, but I feel that they should certainly not be ignored, and, as emotionally-immature, or trouble-making behaviour (witnessing this can drain the life out of someone with my type of nature) is not uncommon on social media, in stark contrast, they stand out hugely in a good light.

As I say: *If something is, it just is.* By that I mean, if someone or something has notable qualities, they do not need vies for attention, as they will be self-evident. I see this all the time when I notice a certain beauty or wonderful quality in others.

We are all aware that there are much unpleasantness and nonsense on social media and parts of it might at times feel as though that is almost all that it is made up of. This is a shame, as there is actually much fabulous, humorous, helpful and heartwarming stuff on there too.

But that particular threatening experience of it, at the time, made me withdraw from the slight progress I had made in getting used to the public aspects that come with being a performer and writer.

17
The Way

B Y NOW, BECAUSE OF RECENT experiences, I had again been put off in showing anything that I might creatively produce. I had previously begun to overcome that but had now reverted back to that state again.

During this time however, my voiceover agent asked me to record a sophisticated-style piece for an international commercial. Something in the script that I was sent made me realise that this was what I enjoyed doing. So, I did the requested recording.

In the end, the commercial was never commissioned due to business-related issues, but regardless, it had been enough to give me the motivation to get back into the studio again and work on bits and pieces of voicing and writing.

But I would continue to struggle to establish my work in that regard, as the situation persisted of being told by the industry professionals that I met the standards and they liked what I could do —with one very high profile entertainments agency being highly enthusiastic about that, which was kind—but all the same they could not commission my work or cast me as a performer, because I was unknown.

Having been scheduled to go to New Zealand to look into relocating over there, despite the painful injuries from the hideous cycling accident that had happened very shortly before (as I had not broken any bones I was still able to fly), I was determined to go ahead with it.

It was almost agonisingly uncomfortable for me at times to fly so far with my physical health issues, but something bizarre, and, according to Ethan, funny, kept happening along the way: I was frequently chatted to by people from various parts of the world who were travelling, who, completely unaware of the physical pain that I was in as I had become adept at hiding it so well, were convinced, for some reason, that I was someone in the public eye, trying to guess among themselves where they apparently recognized me from.

'*Actress from Game of Thrones.*', someone concluded aloud satisfactorily to another, referring to the hit tv programme that I, of course, had never appeared in (or any others for that matter).

When some approached me to try to figure out who I was, I responded by hastily politely explaining that I was not, in fact, known as a person within my industry, or for that matter anyone at all.

It always feels odd and very surprising when such situations arise, as this was one of previous similarly peculiar moments in my life.

But I just found the comments funny. There were many more of them, but some of the sincerity that I was shown bowled me over. It was peculiar to realise that what was now so warmly interpreted as, according to others, likeable about me, was what I had been so often beaten and abused for earlier in my life.

It would be so that later, I would also find myself taken aback at some people in the UK too, being this same very amiable way towards me- why this is I don't know, but it is sweet all the same and I was tickled pink by it.

Often when people had complimented me, they would like to engage me in a quick chat and I was surprised to find that once they got talking to me, they would ask where they might follow my future creative works.

Was it possible that as it turned out from such lovely reactions, that I perhaps should have been seen and heard a little after all? Further, it also seemed possible that because of others kind interest in my qualities, that some might feel a connection with or enjoy some element of that which I could creatively produce. It would later be pointed out to me that it turned out that the features writer from decades earlier, who had playfully said that they had 'discovered' me, had been right about how they felt that the work I could do within the arts and entertainment industries stood a good chance of being enjoyed by audiences and readers. I couldn't believe that I or my prospective work would be liked and that people could be so kind and affectionate towards me. *But would they still feel this way if they knew what I had lived through?*, I wondered, and worried about how they might react to learning about that.

Anyway, back to New Zealand. I felt an instant fondness for the place and its people. I had met good people and seen exceptional places in different parts of the world and here, this was another insightful experience of that kind.

One day, during a contemplative moment, I sat alone amongst lush green trees that swayed in the soft breeze, overlooking one of the vast bays—a stunning sight—glistening in the sunshine. Faced with the rebuilding of my life and the overcoming of my fears about the public aspect of my being a creative artist and performer, given everything that I had lived through, I reflected on what to do about this.

The unfortunate circumstances that had gone against me throughout my life had made it very difficult for me to achieve the things that it was thought that I would go on to do and yet I believed that a lack of serendipity seemed an insufficient reason to not at least *try* to get somewhere.

So, in regard to that earlier question, *was I going to let that experience on social media affect what was left of the life that I had barely ever had the chance to start living properly?*

Well, the thing is, being a victim has never sat at all well with me: I am naturally inclined to instead just get on with my life. I decided that if I gave in to the abuse and threats that I had received on social media from those few particular people, then that would be entering the territory of victim mentality, a way of thinking that I had been at pains to stay away from for all of my life. It is quite simple really; being a victim of something is actually merely a fact or term of reference, but the way that one perceives themselves and their life in relation to that is something entirely different.

Though the violation that I had experienced had affected me, I decided that I had to find the strength to rise above all of that and carry on as best I could with the path that I had originally set off on.

I also did not want others to have their life badly affected as I had. I wanted to show that we can overcome, we can succeed in life, no matter how much we might have given in to our circumstances at one time. In this respect, I began to feel a renewed perspective for what I should do to rebuild my life.

On the way back from New Zealand, a most strange event occurred.

When I, as usual, had to explain my case with the issue of removing my footwear for the security scanners, regarding special requirements for preventing infection when touching the floor, stating that I could only remove my shoes when standing on a clean surface, on this occasion, the security staff did not seem to understand.

Upon noticing the medical compression that I was wearing, along with the combination of my trying to explain the situation regarding my being susceptible to infection with my feet being exposed to the floor, the security personnel appeared to be somewhat suspicious. They sent their female security staff to escort me to a side room for examination.

Unfortunately, the lady spoke very little English, unlike the security staff at the scanners and this language barrier proved to make things a little difficult.

In broken English (nevertheless, her English was perhaps better than my attempt at speaking her language would have been!), the security lady demanded, 'Take legs off.'

I was a little taken aback by this demand and paused in disbelief.

'Take legs off *now*!', said the security lady, with a seeming sense of urgency.

'You want me to...take my legs off?' I echoed with a very puzzled expression.

'Yes, legs off now!' said the lady firmly.

She surely did not mean that, but we were getting lost in translation, as I diplomatically tried to explain.

A couple of armed security personnel now appeared, which began to worry me. Nothing like this had ever happened to me before when travelling. I felt very nervous about this situation but maintained my calm demeanour.

Thankfully though, the security lady seemed at this point to have understood the reason for my disbelief. 'Your legs?' she asked, pointing to my limbs in confusion.

'Yes. My legs,' I replied with a friendly smile, patting my legs. 'Mine.'

It suddenly became apparent that, having never seen compression on the limbs like this before, she either thought that I was wearing prosthetics that could be not what they appeared to be, or that the medical compression garments may have seemed suspicious in some way; it was not clear exactly what it was about them that was causing so much concern, but my medical condition and subsequent requirements were irregular.

The security lady was thorough in feeling my legs and realised that they were, in fact, my own limbs. She continued to pat down my legs and waist, content that she had not found anything of concern, but still seeming confused by the particular compression garments covering my legs and abdomen. 'Why?' the lady asked, pointing up and down at them.

I thought about what I could say: 'cancer', surely, was a universal word? I tried that; it did not work. They could not understand what I was trying to tell them, and, having taken my medical documents away from me, I had nothing now to show them to explain my circumstances.

Fortunately, however, a gentleman who was senior in airport security and spoke very good English came to see what the fuss was about. He enquired with the staff as to what was going on. The man then asked me why I had these very specific medical requirements. Upon my explaining my situation to him, he understood eventually. With this new understanding, they continued further checks, including, this time, my medical documentation.

The head security guy told me that I was now free to go, and I felt a wave of relief come over me at these words.

'I apologise for that,' he said empathetically, 'This is not a regular situation with some of these medical things. May I ask what it is that causes you to need them?'

'When I had cancer treatment, most of my lymph nodes were taken away here.' I pointed at my abdominal area. 'I have lymphoedema, an illness, from that, so the compression garments stop my body from swelling when I fly. But when I am not flying, I do not wear them all the time apart from when exercising.' (Later, I would go on to wear medical compression garments when flying that are embellished with lace, so they just look like pretty lace-top stockings when compression is needed).

Whilst this situation had been more than a little unnerving whilst it was ongoing, nothing awful happened—I was treated courteously, ultimately—and I look back on the whole bizarreness with some amusement; yes, I was once nearly arrested at a major international airport for having had cancer!

Well, being from a most disadvantaged background, but, apparently, with certain qualities, meant that though I always did everything that I could to decline the invitation, I was nevertheless ushered into entry to this strange and surreal party in life; a party which became something of an extravaganza of my unusual circumstances.

Though for sure, for many years, through circumstance, my life was desolate, with those apparently good creative qualities (though I have always felt them to be meagre) that some of the professionals of the arts kindly saw in me throughout my life having to be entirely suppressed. But, indeed, I have never wanted any of my circumstances or experiences to be a reason to lead a depressing life; rather, I am naturally drawn to the interesting, expressive, and bright parts of life.

I cannot deny that I am self-conscious of what I have experienced, and I feel my humanness keenly indeed. But this very humanness is perhaps what enriches my affinity with others. Having lived the kind of life that I have, that comes with a certain understanding of some of the things that people go through, and I want the best for them.

In spite of traumatic experiences—and the overwhelming feelings that can be attached to them for some—our lives absolutely can still have abundant value, purpose and enjoyment.

Even if someone has not been through a particular trauma, I

find that many can sometimes find themselves simply needing to feel rejuvenated, because if life feels disappointing for you or perhaps you might be chasing something that you feel you can never find; love, contentment, peace of mind...?, the possibility of better times ahead is there for you.

Indeed, we can live with and successfully manage our difficulties or sadness whilst enjoying the good parts of life—all the brilliant things that provide us with wonderful antidotes to stress and unpleasantness, however small or fleeting. My love of the arts and nature are some of my essential favourite things in life. My passions are not just about enjoyment; they have got me through many years of pain. I love to learn of others' passions, too. What makes you feel truly alive and at peace?

Although it can feel as though we simply exist sometimes, especially when circumstances prevent us from accessing any true contentment in life, and even perhaps while living with a secret sadness, it is always possible to grow towards a happier life.

Life can at times, be strange and painful, but it is finding what fulfils us within it that makes it all so worthwhile for us.

Hold your values close to your heart and remember what drives you—your loves and your passions—and keep them with you always, even if you are one of those who have had their hopes and dreams beaten down by life.

Whatever your age or circumstances: you may have felt lost, alone, or disheartened, but you will be amazed at how much you can develop yourself as a person even in depressing or frustrating times.

Never lose sight of what makes you feel alive, because, similarly to our intense feelings of pain, discomfort, longing, or frustration, have you ever felt that your heart could burst from sheer joy? Do you remember those little moments and the lovely warm feeling that they gave you? Let's hold onto that feeling.

Is this what that degraded, shy young woman did?

Well, with all the quiet strength and dignity that she could muster, she made the best of her circumstances, stood on her own two feet, overcame and made it through it all.

Epilogue

B Y NOW, I WOULD HAVE liked to have established a body of creative work for the enjoyment of its audience, but unfortunately, circumstances meant that this never happened. Instead, it took several decades for me to receive the opportunity to even be able to begin to contribute anything possibly meaningful as a creative.

To be kindly welcomed into the worlds of film and voiceover as a writer and performer has been a privilege, as it also is if people enjoy my writing, voice and words and performances, and I am tremendously grateful of that.

I have even finally been persuaded to venture into acting professionally, as I was often advised to do all those years ago. I am not sure if it will lead anywhere, but with acting, I am free to express myself creatively and can draw on my various life experiences, so that is where my focus is.

This is a place where I feel at home; a place that had always been there, but which, through sheer misfortune, was always out of my reach, until now.

Those many years of being deprived, threatened and almost hidden away by circumstance, in which I lost out on achieving what I should have done with my life or being able to enjoy living it, I am now beginning to make up for.

You see, though we might feel crushed, sad, and beaten-down by the cruel parts of life, life is actually full of good things—even where and when we would least anticipate it to be so. My mentality, therefore, is, *let's embrace all of the good, comforting, pleasant things in spite of the bad (even if those things are only available in tiny moments).*

Throughout my life, I have known both the very best and, for the overwhelmingly most part, very worst, in human behaviour. I just wish I had seen so much more of the former, for myself and others.

Learning of how I had been conditioned by others to think and feel in certain ways, and coming to realise as such led to my ultimately breaking-free of this. I learned that I simply did not have the tools to do so previously. My mindset has become strengthened in this respect, along with my boundaries.

Now I have established that inner poise that comes from becoming who I always should have been, and I have found a subtle confidence in that.

My spirit may once have almost been entirely broken (*almost* but not actually) by many years of enduring at the hands of those who exerted their power or influence over me, surviving deprivation and abuse from a young age, as well as spending all those years in severe hardship while suffering from serious illness, and those decades it took me to be finally able to begin to establish myself as a creative within the performing arts and entertainment industry. But despite that, my strength of mind is intact, and I use it to make the most of my life.

I hope to reach my ultimate dream of living life as peacefully as possible in a natural environment, and I hope to catch up with you again one day.

And so, here we are, in this story; perhaps a cautionary tale of the pain and devastation that ignorance and arrogance can cause, but despite that, one of how life is for living and that good people are so incredibly worth having a love of life for, even when you might least expect it to be so. Let us never give up hope on that.

But I leave you with one question: where in life do you want to go?

The end?

For me, it is just the beginning...

Acknowledgements

As a reserved person who is generally private, it goes completely against the grain for me to so openly reveal my life experiences, as I have written in this book, which although is not a life story, still feels so against my nature in discussing myself. Indeed, I was almost too afraid to go ahead with the publishing.

However, some in film and publishing, and also some of those in the medical profession, persuaded me that this is a story that has to be told. So, the only way that I could cope with revealing what I had lived through, having been often told that doing so might help to change things for the better for some, was by simply making it part of my work as a writer.

Having lived with the secrets of my experiences for so many years, it took every inch of my courage to write this book, which I wrote by my own hand, but even far more so to allow it to be published despite my intense unease at doing so. This feat is partially thanks to some special people...

Firstly, I dearly thank my husband for standing by me through my treatment for cancer and for his unwavering belief in me and my work as a creative.

Thank you to all of the medical professionals who saved my life and provided the medical care that helped me to overcome the subsequent health problems resulting from the misdiagnosis.

Thanks to my publishing team, with special mention to Hayley and Elise for their considerable patience, trust and understanding throughout the publishing process, and to Mark, for the cover design.

Also, thanks to those in the professional fields of writing, acting, film, voiceover and dance, whom in getting to know me in person had the graciousness to encourage me to show some of my creative works.

My heartfelt love to them all—each and every one.

www.ingramcontent.com/pod-product-compliance
Lightning Source LLC
Chambersburg PA
CBHW051728260326
41914CB00040B/2020/J